The Basics

The Basics is a highly successful series of accessible guidebooks which provide an overview of the fundamental principles of a subject area in a jargon-free and undaunting format.

Intended for students approaching a subject for the first time, the books both introduce the essentials of a subject and provide an ideal springboard for further study. With over 50 titles spanning subjects from artificial intelligence (AI) to women's studies, *The Basics* are an ideal starting point for students seeking to understand a subject area.

Each text comes with recommendations for further study and gradually introduces the complexities and nuances within a subject.

WORLD HISTORY (Second Edition)
Peter N. Stearns

URBAN ANTHROPOLOGY
Julian Brash

ECONOMIC GEOGRAPHY
Julie MacLeavy, Kean Fan Lim, Allan Watson

CHINA
Anna Lora-Wainwright

PUBLIC HEALTH
Fiona Sim and Jenny Wright

For more information about this series, please visit: www.routledge.com/The-Basics/book-series/B

PUBLIC HEALTH
THE BASICS

Fiona Sim and Jenny Wright

Routledge
Taylor & Francis Group
LONDON AND NEW YORK

Designed cover image: Getty Images

First published 2027
by Routledge
4 Park Square, Milton Park, Abingdon, Oxon OX14 4RN

and by Routledge
605 Third Avenue, New York, NY 10158

Routledge is an imprint of the Taylor & Francis Group, an informa business

British Library Cataloguing-in-Publication Data
A catalogue record for this book is available from the British Library

ISBN: 978-1-041-31599-5 (hbk)
ISBN: 978-1-032-83471-9 (pbk)
ISBN: 978-1-003-77990-2 (ebk)

DOI: 10.4324/9781003779902

Typeset in Bembo
by SPi Technologies India Pvt Ltd (Straive)

CONTENTS

ACKNOWLEDGEMENTS

We would like to thank those who have reviewed the book at various stages of its development. We could not have done it without your help.

INTRODUCING PUBLIC HEALTH

Welcome to the world of public health! We are delighted you have decided to find out a bit more about what it means, why it is important, what it aims to achieve and, especially, how it is helping to tackle major health and broader issues of our time. If, by the end, you are moved to join us, we will show you how you, too, might contribute. We would emphasise that the book is written from a UK base but, where useful and appropriate, has information and examples from other countries.

The goal of the public health movement, and of those who work within it, is to improve health and prevent disease for people, not only individuals but crucially groups of people, whole communities or populations. This is an enormous task which we will try to make sense of. If we say, for example, 'public health is good in this area', that is shorthand for saying 'the population in the area is healthy, people live in an environment that helps to keep them that way, there are few preventable premature (early) deaths and anyone who needs health or social care is able to access the services from which they can benefit'. This comment is often placed in the context of a comparison with other areas. It should be the norm for all of us in the United Kingdom (UK), though it is often seen as a Utopian dream and 'good' is not always attainable as we shall see.

Historically, public health was mainly concerned with the detection and management of infectious diseases. Today, however, in the UK and similar countries, the scope is much broader with early public health measures having tackled major issues such as ensuring everyone has access to clean water and childhood immunisation. As medicine has advanced and health needs have changed, so too

DOI: 10.4324/9781003779902-1

has public health developed for the modern era. In nineteenth-century England, for example, the average life expectancy at birth was around 40 years. By 2023, it had risen in the UK to 79 years for men and 83 years for women for the period 2021 to 2023.[1]

Whereas in the nineteenth century, public health achievements were linked to improved sanitation and controlling infectious diseases, in the twentieth century, as overall health in the population improved, attention shifted to improving health services and reducing other huge, preventable threats to health such as those posed by smoking. Today, we are more aware of the issues which have an impact on both our physical and mental health such as climate change, air quality, access to health and social care, poverty, being physically active, tackling obesity and poor nutrition. The public health workforce aims to help tackle all these real-world issues. In doing this, they intersect with other aspects of people's lives such as government, the economy and respect for human rights.

Before we move on, let us just explain a way in which the term 'public health' is used which might cause substantial confusion. It is when the public health workforce is described as 'public health'. For example, you might read about the responsibilities or achievements of public health, when it is the workforce that is being described and not the health of the population served by that workforce. Throughout this book, to prevent this confusion, we shall try to use terms including 'public health workforce', 'public health people', 'public health practitioners/specialists/team' or even 'public health movement' to describe the human effort involved in the endeavour to improve the health of a population. Please be aware of this ambiguity in commonly used terminology in your outside reading.

Another ambiguity is that in some countries, although not in the UK, 'public health' may be used to describe publicly funded healthcare provision. It is worth being aware of this, too.

Although many more people than before have some understanding of public health as a result of the COVID-19 pandemic, nevertheless it can remain a subject that is remote and difficult to access. As an entity – or sometimes a movement – that is simply all about the health of a particular population or community, it should be readily accessible. However, as a discipline that sees itself both as an *art* and a *science* and which sometimes appears to be influenced by contemporary mores and politics as much as the strength of its evidence base, it can seem complicated.

There are numerous definitions of 'public health'. In 1948, the World Health Organization (WHO, part of the United Nations system[2]) described health as 'a state of complete physical, mental and social well-being and not merely the absence of disease or infirmity' and that 'public health refers to all organized measures (whether public or private) to prevent disease, promote health, and prolong life among the population as a whole. Its activities aim to provide conditions in which people can be healthy and focus on populations, not on individual patients or diseases.'[3]

The emphasis here, therefore, is on *population* not *individual* health and this is what distinguishes public health from the classic practice of clinical medicine where the focus is on the individual patient. Looking at the population's health can apply to the whole population or specific groups within the population such as older people, children, specific ethnic groups – in the UK, for example, the risk of type 2 diabetes appears to be higher in people of South Asian origin than in other ethnic groups.[4]

The definition of public health that has been in common usage in the UK for a few decades now is the one proposed in 1988 by Sir Donald Acheson, the Chief Medical Officer at the time: 'the science and art of preventing disease, prolonging life and promoting health through the organised efforts of society'.[5] In 2004, Sir Derek Wanless, an English banker and adviser to the Labour Government, broadened Acheson's notion of society when he defined public health as 'the science and art of preventing disease, prolonging life and promoting health through the organised efforts *and informed choices of society, organisations, public and private, communities and individuals*'.[6]

These definitions emphasise that there is *science* behind public health, and we will see in subsequent sections what this means in terms of mapping and understanding disease in populations including the strong evidence base which underpins our work. It also emphasises the *art* of public health which relates to the wider skills of communication, engagement of individuals, communities, organisations and governments, who all have a role to play in health. This, too, will be explored later in the book.

The WHO, in a later vision for public health, included the aim to reduce (health) *inequalities*. This adds a focus, as we shall see, which underpins much public health activity today.

In defining public health, and in striving to improve it, we must always remember the wider factors that can affect health. Göran

Dahlgren and Margaret Whitehead, public health academics from the University of Liverpool, produced a model in 1991 of the different factors influencing health which included elements such as education, work, the conditions we live in alongside what we are born with. It has been much copied and built upon since.

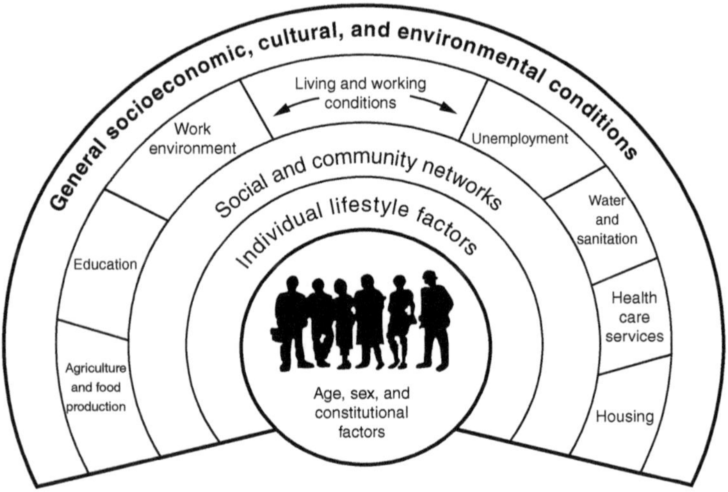

Source: Dahlgren, G. and Whitehead, *M. Policies and Strategies to Promote Social Equity in Health*, Stockholm, Sweden: Institute for Futures Studies

Many people who work in public health are driven by a sense of *social justice*, a desire to make the world – or a little part of it – a better place. Public health is, however, a *collective endeavour*. The workforce has to be prepared, therefore, to be flexible, adaptable and work alongside those whose help they need to secure their goals. This could be at international, national, regional, or local levels and with a variety of different organisations, (such as government, local councils, community groups) and different structures. It is essential to engage with representatives of the population themselves to appreciate their own priorities including their goals for public health: solutions are often co-designed with them.

Because of the longstanding nature of many problems threatening health and the complexity of dealing with issues such as tobacco control, climate change, obesity, it often takes a long time to see results.

The risks from smoking, for example, were first known about in the 1950s.[7] Legislation to restrict advertising began slowly in the UK in the 1960s, but smoking in public places was not banned until 2005/6. Therefore, those working in public health must be both determined and patient. Frequently, government support and legislation are required, and this takes the public health workforce into the realm of public policy, requiring resilience, negotiation and facilitation skills to weather the ups and downs on the road to achieving positive change.

Collaborative working or working in partnership with other people, organisations and across sectors is a hallmark of what works in public health and of what determines a community's health and wellbeing. Perhaps surprisingly for readers just setting out to understand public health, the National Health Service (NHS), while an indispensable feature of British society, is often a minor player or, in some instances, hardly involved at all, in initiatives for improving or protecting the health of a population. For many interventions, for example local authority environmental health services to ensure food safety, local government is more relevant than healthcare. Given that the main determinants of health and of health inequalities lie outside of healthcare, many of the ways of improving health and preventing ill health also sit outside the NHS.

The *social gradient*, whereby people living in more affluent areas are generally found to live longer and be in better health than people living in less affluent areas, is influenced by household income, which has little directly to do with the NHS.[8] The healthcare system is unlikely to be able to influence household income, but public health evidence shows clearly that the whole population would be both healthier and more economically productive if fewer people lived in poverty.

Against international comparisons, income inequality is very marked in the UK.[9] The Marmot Review of 2010 highlighted the substantial gap between the incomes of the richest and poorest in society.[10] A later report in 2022 not only showed this difference had an adverse impact on life expectancy but that the gap had widened since 2010.[11] At central government and at local level, therefore, policies that increase household income among the least well off in society are actually public health actions. Increases in taxation that result in reduced population level consumption of harmful products, such as alcohol and tobacco, may also be described as public health measures. It is crucially important that governments look upstream to tackle the causes of poor health.

Throughout this book, you will find examples where the solution to a public health issue might look simple or relatively easy to implement but in reality, is complicated, time-consuming, fraught with either anticipated or unexpected opposition, and involves many organisations and people.

This book is here to help dispense myths, explain in straightforward language and show the importance of public health as well as present the challenges. Where appropriate, we will present examples to illustrate practice.

Public health is a complex subject which we have aimed to condense into manageable chapters to make it more accessible to the reader. The reader can dip into the different Parts and Chapters, depending on interest, or read the book straight through. The book is divided into three main parts and each part into chapters relating to a particular topic:

- PART 1
  Development and evolution of public health from the mid nineteenth century
- PART 2
  Demystifying public health
- PART 3
  Challenges to health

This is not a textbook nor a comprehensive coverage of such a vast topic, but an introductory reader intended to inform and inspire, but also to present the realities of the challenges we all face. We hope you will enjoy finding out more.

NOTES

1 Life expectancy in England for males at birth in 1841 was 40 years and 42 for females. The more recent figures are still below pre-pandemic levels. https://www.ons.gov.uk/peoplepopulationandcommunity/birthsdeathsandmarriages/lifeexpectancies/articles/howhaslifeexpectancychangedovertime/2015-09-09; https://www.ons.gov.uk/peoplepopulationandcommunity/birthsdeathsandmarriages/lifeexpectancies/bulletins/nationallifetablesunitedkingdom/2021to2023additionaldata

2 WHO is a specialised agency of the United Nations which coordinates responses to international public health issues and emergencies.
3 Who.int/about/governance/constitution
4 Perhaps partly explained by people of South Asian heritage being more likely than others to store fat around their middles (visceral fat) which increases the risk of developing type 2 diabetes at lower levels of BMI. https://www.diabetes.org.uk/node/12895
5 Acheson, D. *Public Health in England: Report of the Committee of Inquiry into the Future Development of the Public Health Function*, Cm 289, HMSO, 1988.
6 Wanless, D. *Securing Good Health for the Whole Population, Final Report*, London, HMSO, 25 February 2004.
7 A prospective study of doctors' smoking habits by Sir Richard Doll and Sir Austin Bradford Hill showed that there was a strong association between smoking and lung cancer and also between smoking and cardiovascular disease. Although there were only 36 lung cancer deaths in the first 29 months of the study, after four years there were 200, almost all of them in heavy smokers. The incidence in non-smokers was negligible. Doll and Hill began publishing their results in the *BMJ* in 1954 (Doll, R. and Bradford Hill, A., 'The Mortality of Doctors in Relation to their Smoking Habits', *BMJ* 1954;228(i): 1451–5).
8 In countries without universal healthcare provision, then, of course, access to healthcare and the provision of healthcare is influenced directly by household income.
9 https://ifs.org.uk/articles/income-and-wealth-inequality-explained-5-charts
10 Marmot, M., Goldblatt, P., Allen, J. et al. *Fair Society, Healthy Lives (the Marmot Review)*, Institute of Health Equity, February 2010.
11 In 2022, a report from the King's Fund explained that in England, there is a systematic relationship between deprivation and life expectancy. In 2017–19, women living in the least-deprived 10 per cent of areas could, at birth, expect to live to 86.4 years old, whereas women in the most-deprived 10 per cent of areas could expect to live to 78.7 years – a gap in life expectancy of almost 8 years. For men, this gap was even wider, with a difference of 9.4 years between the life expectancy for those in the least-deprived 10 per cent of areas (83.5 years) and the most-deprived 10 per cent of areas (74.1 years). In recent years, inequalities in life expectancy by deprivation have widened. https://www.kingsfund.org.uk/insight-and-analysis/long-reads/what-are-health-inequalities

PART 1

DEVELOPMENT AND EVOLUTION OF PUBLIC HEALTH FROM THE MID NINETEENTH CENTURY

INTRODUCTION

We will give a historical perspective to public health and some context to help explain the ways that current challenges to health are being tackled. This part of the book will show the complexity of population health issues and how different countries, over the years, have responded to changing health problems. We will also touch on the workforces recruited to help deliver programmes to improve health. This will be explored in more detail in Part 2, Chapter 6.

Our main focus will be on chronological developments from the middle of the nineteenth century when the governments of countries, principally in the Western World (Great Britain, Western Europe, North America, Australia and New Zealand), made concerted efforts to tackle perceived harms to human health. That is not to say that previous societies had not made efforts. The Romans brought clean water to their cities separately from sanitary waste systems. Medieval societies, and even earlier ones, used quarantine measures and isolation of diseased individuals, to protect themselves in times of plague or leprosy.

It is the nineteenth century, however, that we turn to for the start of the modern public health era. It was then that we saw the beginnings of collective action against disease. Most of this early response aimed to deal with health problems stemming from the rapid development of towns and cities following large scale industrialisation.

DOI: 10.4324/9781003779902-2

In the Western World this occurred from 1830s. For many other countries, rapid industrialisation only happened after the Second World War and was, for some, linked to the end of colonial empires.

Part 1 is not an exhaustive account. Rather, it is designed to give a broad overview of significant changes and their impact on population health, with some illustrative examples drawn from different countries and time periods.

The history of modern public health can be divided into different phases:

- sanitary health, when effort went into providing clean water and sewerage systems;
- scientific approaches following the discovery of the cause and means of transmission of many infectious diseases;
- preventive measures with a focus on maternal and child welfare;
- the promise of clinical medicine and of better health and social care;
- the adverse effects of modern environments on people's health leading to the need for different approaches including behaviour change (sometimes described as the 'new' public health)

As we shall see, each change was accompanied by debate, controversy and resistance. Societies addressed tackling threats to population health according to their own experience, cultures, history, and political structures.

The outline for Part 1 is as follows:

- the modern public health era in the Western World
- public health in low- and middle-income countries (LMICs)
- international and global approaches to public health

1

THE EMERGENCE OF THE MODERN PUBLIC HEALTH ERA IN THE WESTERN WORLD

1. SANITARY HEALTH AND THE SOCIAL REFORM FROM THE MIDDLE OF THE NINETEENTH CENTURY

I) GREAT BRITAIN

a) Impact of industrialisation

Before industrialisation, societies were mainly based on agriculture with small industries using hand production methods. The transition to mechanised production from 1750 involved steam and water-power, with new chemical manufacturing and iron production processes. This development was preceded by changes in agricultural methods from the middle of the seventeenth century. These included moving to a four-course rotation of crops,[1] which increased land productivity and to selective breeding of cattle. Both served to increase food supply. Along with a population explosion in the eighteenth century stemming from a fall in mortality,[2] many people in country areas were freed to move to cities where they were needed to man the new factories.

Britain was the first industrialised nation in the world. The population of towns and cities grew rapidly from the end of the eighteenth century. London, for example, doubled its population between 1801 and 1831,[3] leading to insufficient housing and gross overcrowding in slum areas surrounding the new factories.

DOI: 10.4324/9781003779902-3

In Liverpool, 30,000 people lived in cellars in the 1840s.[4] Inadequate sewerage systems and infrequent refuse collection meant filth was merely dumped in streets and outside houses. The stench was appalling. Death rates rose.

Several influences were in play to bring about change. The first was the belief that people's health was a matter of public concern. In the nineteenth century, this stemmed from humanitarians'[5] desire to help the less fortunate members of society, as seen in moves to abolish slavery and the slave trade. Some businessmen also contributed. John Cadbury, for example, built Bournville village in Birmingham to ensure workers had better living conditions. Alongside these humanitarian motives was the practical need to have a fit population to work in factories and meet the demands of expanding trade. However, it was the high death toll from a wave of cholera epidemics, reaching Britain from Europe in 1831, which finally led to definitive action. This took the form of investigations into data on deaths and on the working and living conditions of the poor. William Farr, a physician who pioneered the quantitative study of mortality (deaths) and morbidity (illness),[6] joined the General Register Office in 1837 from where he analysed statistics about cause of death. He also used Census[7] data to refine indicators for overcrowding, publishing evidence on preventable disease in industrial cities.[8]

b) The beginnings of social reform

Edwin Chadwick, a lawyer committed to social reform, as Secretary of the Poor Law Commission,[9] was concerned about the costs of disease to society, which, by causing incapacity to work, interfered with economic efficiency. His investigations in East London led to his *Report on the Sanitary Conditions of the Labouring Population of Great Britain* in 1842. Chadwick, like Farr, associated disease with filth. This was in accordance with the prevailing miasma theory[10] that diseases such as cholera were caused by bad (noxious) air coming from rotting organic matter. They thought, therefore, that disease was due to filthy environmental conditions such as lack of drainage, no clean water supply or means of removing rubbish from houses and streets. Although their solution was beneficial to health, by focusing on bad sanitation as the cause of disease, Chadwick's ideas, nevertheless, could be criticised for deflecting attention from other potent influences such as malnutrition and poverty.

Chadwick's Public Health Act of 1848 was a pragmatic response to insanitary conditions in large cities. It empowered the Central Board of Health to establish local boards with powers to deal with water supply and sewerage (sanitary reform). Liverpool, where conditions were particularly bad following the arrival of many thousands of Irish peasants fleeing famine, had passed its own Sanitary Act in 1846. This gave the council authority to appoint a Medical Officer of Health (MOH) to oversee sanitary improvements. Following the 1848 Act, more cities began to appoint their own MOsH. Urban water supplies did start to improve but sanitation was expensive and its implementation slow. There was also some resistance to state intervention. *The Times*, for example, stated in its editorial on 1 August 1854 that 'We prefer to take our chance with cholera than be bullied into health.' Rate payers were also not happy to have local taxes raised.

The subsequent Public Health Act of 1875 divided the country into urban and rural sanitary districts, each subject to supervision by a Local Government Board. It became mandatory for each district to have a MOH whose primary role was oversight of provision to improve the health of the community. This merger of local government with public health transformed the concept of health. Public health came to be equated to whatever the local board did to improve the environment for its citizens. This might include wide streets and the provision of park land as well as water and sewerage systems, all seen as contributing to the 'physical, moral and mental health' of the population.

Working conditions in factories also came under the spotlight. Of particular concern were the long hours worked in unsanitary conditions, accidents due to unprotected machines and lack of ventilation. The first Factory Act of 1833 in England protected child labour, forbidding employment under the age of nine in textile factories. A system of factory inspection was established. The Mines and Collieries Act of 1842 prohibited the employment of women and boys under the age of ten underground whereas the Factory Act of 1850 fixed the working day for women and children in textile mills between 6am and 6pm, with an hour and a half for meals. Later Factory Acts in the 1860s extended the range of industries covered to include potteries, matches, hosiery lace, iron, copper and brass foundries.[11] All of these Acts were preceded by agitation and public inquiries and were fiercely opposed by many employers.

II) SANITARY REFORM IN WESTERN EUROPE

Industrialisation came slightly later in other countries in Western Europe, which were subject to periodic revolutions and structural reform. They, nevertheless, followed Britain's lead in undertaking sanitary reforms, although implementation was at times piecemeal, depending on the nature of each country's governing structure.

a) France

From the 1830s, France created its first heavy industries and migration to cities led to similar problems of overcrowding as in Britain. One of the main social reformers was the economist and physician, Louis-Rene Villerme. He collected information, using the '*méthode numérique*', on deaths in the poorer districts in Paris and made associations between these and environmental factors. His 1840 report on the health conditions of textile workers led to the regulation of child labour in factories. Unlike Britain, however, there was no national state response to urban problems and the main protagonists for change were social and medical activists. The French Revolution of 1789 had included health in the Declaration of the Rights of Man but also the sanctity of private property and individual liberty. The State was wary, therefore, of any interventions that might lead to popular resistance, with the result that actions to improve sanitation only took place at the local level. Following the 1832 cholera epidemic in Paris, for example, it was *The Globe* newspaper that proposed that the city be provided with an adequate supply of good water and a proper sewerage system.

b) Germany

Industrialisation had similar impacts on urban dwelling in Germany. Until unification in 1871, Germany was a collection of nation states of which Prussia was the largest. Agitation for sanitary reform came mainly from a group of medical men, led by Rudolf Virchow, a physician, pathologist, anthropologist and politician, known to his colleagues as the 'pope of medicine'. This group believed the health of the people was a matter of social concern and that society had an obligation to protect the health of its members. Sanitary reform did not take place, however, until after unification and remained the responsibility of constituent Federal States.[12] The central Reich Health Office was only responsible for statistics collection, infectious disease control and smallpox vaccination.

c) Sweden

Sweden's story is different again. In the eighteenth century, the government, wanting to increase its productive workforce to support the country's economic expansion, put in place a programme for medical care with public assistance for the sick, poor and disabled. Industrialisation did not take place until the very end of the nineteenth century. Until then, most of the population remained in agricultural occupations. However, Sweden was not immune to the wave of epidemics and infectious diseases crippling the rest of Europe from the 1830s. This led to the establishment in 1862 of local Boards of Health responsible for sanitary reform as well as the district medical officers and epidemic hospitals.

Most of the southern and eastern European states (including Spain, Italy, Greece, Yugoslavia, Poland) did not address sanitary problems stemming from dense urban living until the early twentieth century.

III) SANITARY REFORM IN FRONTIER SOCIETIES AND IMPACT ON INDIGENOUS POPULATIONS

The introduction of sanitary reform in countries settled by migrants from Europe followed a different trajectory. These countries were highly protective of the idea of individual liberty and resistant to imposition of reforms from national institutions. Public health action was, therefore, localised. In the United States of America, for example, as in France, health was seen as a right of citizens, but it was the citizens' own responsibility to maintain their health.

a) United States

The United States was, of course, subject to the effects, as elsewhere, of rapid urbanisation and of epidemics of communicable diseases fuelled by waves of migration. There was no central control. The

American Public Health Association,[13] founded in 1872, welcomed membership from disciplines including medicine, science, public health administration, government and social reform. It contributed reports on the state of sanitary conditions in major cities. New York, Boston and Chicago invested in municipal water and sanitation projects because of the impacts of overcrowding and disease, aided by pressure from social reformers such as Benjamin McCready, Lemuel Shattuck and John Griscom[14] who had been influenced by the work of Chadwick (UK) and Villerme (France). As late as 1875, many large US cities did not have a health department. There was no national coordination. A National Board of Health set up from 1879 to 1883 applied quarantine regulations between States after a disastrous yellow fever epidemic in the Mississippi Valley. The imposition of the Reservation System[15] on Native Americans from the 1830s to the 1870s meant also the imposition of vaccination, fumigation and quarantine measures, but overcrowded living conditions led to a high incidence of tuberculosis (TB).

b) Canada

It was a similar story in Canada. The British North America Act of 1867 created the Dominion of Canada through a confederation of four Provinces. Ontario was the first provincial government to establish a Board of Health in 1882. This provided a model for other Provinces. These Boards only operated in times of epidemics to supervise special measures. The settler Canadians were mainly concerned to ensure there were treatment facilities in place should they fall ill. There was a belief that the bracing northern climate purified the environment and thus afforded settlers special protection. Strategies to limit the spread of infection met with resistance and were regarded as interfering. The Federal Government had to confine its role to screening and quarantining people arriving from abroad. Industrialisation came at the end of the nineteenth century, affecting the largest towns where rapid population growth resulting from immigration made conditions worse. Sanitary reform, principally led by voluntary organisations and social reformers advocating better hygiene, was left to individual cities and Provinces to legislate for and manage. Communicable diseases brought by settlers took a particularly heavy toll on the indigenous population, although a campaign to vaccinate all Native people against smallpox did take place in the early twentieth century.[16]

c) Australia and New Zealand

Australia and New Zealand were also slow to adopt effective public health legislation and sanitary measures. This stemmed from the independent approach of a frontier society plus the belief that the 'colonies' were naturally healthier away from the Old World and little was needed in the way of legislation. British colonisation of Australia had begun with the transportation of British convicts from the end of the eighteenth century and of New Zealand from 1840, when Maori chiefs ceded land to the British crown. Conditions for the working classes in cities were poor, with frequent epidemics of typhoid. A further problem was that these countries needed to attract investment for their development. Therefore, they down-played health issues or blamed them on the habits and morals of the poor. As in the USA and Canada, the indigenous populations were vulnerable to imported infectious diseases introduced by European migrants and many died. As in North America, residential reserves were created to contain the indigenous Aboriginal population who continued to live in poor conditions.

2. DEVELOPMENT OF PUBLIC HEALTH MEASURES FOR THE PREVENTION OF DISEASE

It was not long before the next phase of public health development came into being. The miasma theory of disease causation, upon which nineteenth-century social reformers based their rationale for environmental change, had been founded on flawed science. Debates raged over the causes and transmission of disease – was it something in the air, an individual's personal makeup, could it pass from person to person? As the century progressed, scientific advances shed new light on both the causes of infectious diseases and how they were transmitted. This enabled the public health agenda to move from sanitation to prevention, as doctors became able to define infectious diseases, monitor them accurately and eventually provide an effective intervention. There was, nevertheless, scepticism about scientific advances, based on religion, societal beliefs, culture, or threats to existing professions. These frequently delayed acceptance in adopting new scientific knowledge.

I) LEARNING TO PREVENT SCURVY AND SMALLPOX

Some scientific advances had been made in the eighteenth century to treat scurvy which we now know is caused by deficiency of Vitamin C. In 1747, James Lind, a Scottish doctor, carried out an early clinical trial and epidemiological investigation on scurvy among sailors on long voyages. He developed a hypothesis, designed a study and then observed and tested six study groups and published the results which suggested that citrus fruits – now known to contain vitamin C – successfully treated sailors with scurvy. Lemon or lime juice was eventually introduced from 1800 to prevent or treat scurvy in sailors on long voyages.

There were also already measures to limit the spread and harm from smallpox. Variolation, the early form of vaccination by a technique which used material from the pustules of a smallpox patient to inoculate uninfected people against the disease, was used in China from the tenth century. It reached Turkey in the seventeenth century. It was not introduced to England until 1721 by Lady Mary Wortley Montagu, the wife of the British Ambassador to Constantinople and a respected writer of travelogues. She had smallpox herself in 1715, survived and, wishing to protect her children, had her son age five inoculated. On her return to England in 1721, she had her daughter inoculated. The Princess of Wales was so impressed she had her own daughters inoculated in 1722. From Britain, variolation was widely adopted across Western Europe and in North America.

A much less risky method of preventing smallpox, using material from cowpox, a disease of cattle that we now know is caused by a similar virus, was established following the work of Edward Jenner, an English physician and scientist. In 1756 he discovered that it was possible to inoculate a person with cowpox material which then made them immune to smallpox. This was based on the same principle as variolation, that is, giving an individual a mild case of the disease had a protective effect. By 1800, inoculation was adopted by the British armed forces and the practice spread to Europe, North America and the British Empire.

A Swiss canton was the first State to make inoculation against smallpox compulsory in 1806. Free vaccination for smallpox was made available in Britain through the Poor Law medical services from 1840. It became compulsory in Britain in 1853 for all infants within their first three months of life and, from 1867, there were penalties for parents who did not comply.

The cowpox virus was used as a natural vaccine until the twentieth century when a modern smallpox vaccine was developed. More recently, a newer modified virus has been used to create a vaccine to prevent the spread of monkeypox, now called Mpox.

II) GERM THEORY AND THE CAUSATION OF CERTAIN DISEASES

The miasma theory of disease causation first came under serious threat through the work of John Snow, an anaesthetist, working in London and credited as one of the founders of modern epidemiology. He provided the earliest epidemiological basis for the 'modern' theory of contagion.[17] He looked at the distribution of 500 deaths in Soho during a ten-day period of a cholera epidemic in 1854 and found the highest rates were in people who lived close to, or used, a water pump in Broad Street. Brewery workers, who drank mostly beer rather than water, and poor residents in the area who fetched water from separate – and it turned out – uncontaminated wells escaped the epidemic. The final clue was a widow in Hampstead who died of cholera despite being nowhere near the 'bad air' of Soho – her servant had fetched her a bottle of water from the Broad Street pump every day. Snow concluded the pump was contaminated and persuaded the authorities to remove the handle. In 1855, he published his views on the cause and spread of cholera due to drinking water contaminated by the excreta of cholera patients discharged into the River Thames. He also showed that cholera could be transmitted from person to person through soiled hands.

Following Snow's work, William Budd, a physician working in Bristol, confirmed, through epidemiological investigations, that drinking water was also the vehicle of transmission of typhoid fever. He found that 'poisons' involved in infectious diseases multiplied in the intestines of sick people and were present in faeces. His investigations into the spread of typhoid among people who had attended a ball found that they had been served water from a well close to where a typhoid sufferer's excreta were deposited.

Despite a lack of firm proof, 'germ' theory started to gain ground in scientific circles. Germ theorists (correctly as we now know) believed that micro-organisms, known as pathogens or germs, could cause disease and could be transmitted from person to person or by contact with sewage or contaminated food or water.

III) THE DEVELOPMENT OF VACCINATION

Louis Pasteur, a French chemist, pharmacist and microbiologist, was responsible for establishing the principles of microbial[18] fermentation and pasteurisation and for demonstrating the potential of immunisation using a less virulent strain of the pathogenic microbes. He wrote about the germ theory of disease but was not able to prove it until he was asked, in the late 1860s, to look at two diseases in silkworms which were ruining the French silk industry. His research concluded that living micro-organisms were the cause. He also studied the process of fermentation in milk, beer and wine and found that bad fermentation was due to contamination with disease-causing microbes in the atmosphere. He showed that one way to destroy these was by heating the liquid – thus inventing the process we call pasteurisation. When he published his theory that the micro-organisms which contaminated liquids also floated in the air he was met with ridicule from the medical establishment.

Definitive proof of germ theory, however, had to wait until the development of sophisticated microscopes to isolate and examine microscopic organisms. These were not available until near the end of the nineteenth century.[19] Robert Koch, a German rural district medical officer, one of the founders of modern medicine and microbiology, was able to use the new microscopes to build on Pasteur's work and, by growing bacteria, prove that specific microbes caused disease. In 1876, he showed that anthrax was transmissible, that it was capable of being passed from one animal to another, and that the disease was caused by the anthrax bacillus[20]. He then went on to identify different bacteria causing septicaemia (1878), tuberculosis (TB) (1882), and cholera (1883). He provided, in other words, a scientific basis for how communicable diseases impact the public's health. Koch and Pasteur, two of the greatest figures in microbiology and in getting germ theory accepted, were great rivals, not helped by the tense relationship at the time between France and Germany. Pasteur was working in Strasbourg when Alsace-Lorraine was seized by Germany.

By the end of the nineteenth century, the causal organisms of several other diseases had also been discovered – typhoid, leprosy diphtheria, dysentery, plague – as well as the link between mosquitoes and malaria and yellow fever and the role of animal vectors[21] as intermediaries in the spread of certain communicable disease.

In the mid-1860s, Joseph Lister, a British surgeon, influenced by Pasteur's work, applied germ theory to prevent wound infection in patients whilst working in Glasgow thereby pioneering aseptic[22] surgery. He advocated chemical disinfection – carbolic acid – to sterilise surgical instruments, patients' skin, sutures and surgeons' hands, thereby introducing the principle of antisepsis.[23]

Louis Pasteur proceeded to do further work towards the end of the nineteenth century to establish the principle of prophylactic (preventive) inoculation. He thought that if inoculation could be developed for smallpox, then it could be produced for other diseases. He prepared material using artificially weakened strains of bacteria starting with cholera in chickens and anthrax in cows, a process he called 'vaccination'.[24] In the 1880s he produced the first vaccine for rabies.

Following Pasteur's work, Emile von Behring, a German physiologist, developed a vaccine against diphtheria in 1894 for which he became known as the 'saviour of children' and for which he was awarded the Nobel Prize in 1901.

These developments paved the way for human vaccines for bacterial infections such as cholera, plague and typhoid and, in the twentieth century, for TB, and then for viral diseases including yellow fever and poliomyelitis (polio). At the same time, scientists discovered that the blood of animals and people who had been immunised or who had recovered from an infection, contained proteins called antibodies. These destroyed invading organisms and blood containing such antibodies was found to have therapeutic and preventive properties when injected into other people who were infected or at very high risk from infection.

IV) IMPROVED MANAGEMENT OF INFECTIOUS DISEASES

These developments on the continent meant that, at the end of the nineteenth century, John Simon, Medical Officer to the General Board of Health in England, could show, through reliable statistics, that people with an infectious disease who remained in the community without being isolated, spread their disease. He considered it would be better, therefore, if a range of major diseases was made compulsorily notifiable and ill people isolated. This led to the Infectious Disease (Notification) Act of 1899 covering smallpox, diphtheria, typhoid and smallpox. This law is still in existence today with over 30 diseases currently mandatorily notifiable in the UK.[25] Doctors remain obliged to report these diseases to public health authorities when diagnosed.

The way was open to more specific control of communicable diseases through effective diagnosis and management by specialist doctors and laboratory scientists. The United States was among the first to establish bacteriological laboratories to diagnose infectious diseases among incoming boat passengers following the 1891 Immigration Act. In 1912, the United States Public Health Service was formed and authorised to investigate TB, hookworm, malaria and leprosy and deal with sanitation, water supplies and sewage disposal. France also had a corps of regional inspectors of hygiene services from 1888 at city council level, supported by laboratories and disinfection services set up to combat infectious diseases.

In Canada, Ontario established their first public health laboratory in 1890. Bacteriological laboratories were then established in other provinces to check milk and water supplies, test suspected diphtheria and typhoid samples and investigate rabies outbreaks.

There was still a degree of resistance to the principle of mass immunisation. Beyond smallpox, countries were slow to introduce routine immunisation programmes. France's first public health law in 1902 combined sanitation measures with compulsory immunisation against some diseases. Immunisation of school children against smallpox was introduced in the United States in the 1920s. In Britain, diphtheria immunisation was introduced in the early 1940s. Routine immunisation programmes for children for the prevention of pertussis, poliomyelitis and TB were not introduced until the 1950s. The UK Public Health Act of 1936 permitted compulsory detaining and treating of patients with TB in the UK. Mobile X-ray units were in place to detect pulmonary (lung) TB from the 1940s, then retained through the introduction of the NHS until being phased out by the 1980s.

3. THE SOCIAL HYGIENE ERA

I) TACKLING POOR GENERAL HEALTH THROUGH WELFARE INITIATIVES, PRIMARILY FOR CHILDREN AND MOTHERS

The developments in immunology and microbiology at the end of the nineteenth century had led to the discovery of the causes of many infectious diseases, the development of new vaccines, antisepsis for surgery and wound treatment and, in Britain, government intervention in public health for disease monitoring. By 1900, deaths from infectious disease in Western Europe and the United States had declined, a fall which had started before, but which was aided by, the bacteriological discoveries. Whilst bacteriology could diagnose certain diseases, it did not have the capability to treat or prevent them. Moreover, despite the provision of basic, clean water and sewage disposal facilities and improvements to the physical environment in the sanitation era, in the drive to combat waves of epidemics, the health of poorer populations still lagged behind the health of more affluent people.

Attitudes, therefore, needed to change. The Boer War in the early twentieth century for Britain, and, later, the First World War for other European countries, exposed the lack of fitness of men for military service. Likewise, the Spanish-American war over Cuba in 1898, in which ten times more men died from disease than from battle, led to recognition in the United States, that more attention needed to be paid to the general health of its population. Public health at the start of the twentieth century needed, therefore, to broaden its scope.

Charles Booth, a British shipowner who was also a social researcher and reformer, prepared innovative philanthropic studies on working class life. In 1902, he wrote *Life and Labour of the People of London* presenting statistics he had collected on poverty in the East End. He demonstrated the extent that people suffered from malnutrition, poor health and lack of physical fitness. The number of maternal deaths was high as were the numbers of still births and of children dying in their first year of life (infant mortality). He highlighted a gross inequality in the distribution of wealth, which we now recognise as a key determinant of inequalities in health.

Britain was not alone in exposing the impact of poor working conditions and the health effects of poverty, unhealthy living conditions and lack of general hygiene, adequate maternity and postnatal[26] care and bad nutrition. The response across the Western World was a suite of welfare initiatives aimed at tackling infant mortality, much of which it was believed could be prevented. Actions included providing clean milk, educating mothers in particular, in the safe care of children, setting up clinics for pregnant women and school medical inspections. Breast feeding was encouraged to avoid the risk of using contaminated milk. Nurseries were provided where babies of working mothers could be left safely. In the United States the Rockefeller Foundation established model programmes emphasising education and prevention. As in the UK, the focus was on encouraging personal responsibility through education although this was tinged with an element of blame.

Canada commenced initiatives to protect maternal and child health in the 1920s alongside immunisation programmes and pasteurisation legislation. However, implementation was met with resistance from the medical profession, fearing interference with their private practice. There was similar hostility in Australia and New Zealand to the imposition of State maternity clinics

II) THE START OF FORMAL PUBLIC HEALTH PROGRAMMES IN GREAT BRITAIN

In Britain, public health nursing was developed initially by local authorities and voluntary associations. The work of these nurses was directed at schools, maternal and child health, and the control of TB.

Health visiting began in Manchester. In 1862, the Ladies Section of the Manchester and Salford Sanitary Association began to employ 'respectable women' to do house to house visits to teach families about health and hygiene in the poorer areas of town. Formal training requirements were established after the Maternity and Child Welfare Act of 1918 and health visitors became part of the local government-based public health service at the time of the First World War (1914–18).[27]

School medical inspection was introduced on a national scale in England in 1907 when a medical department was created at the Board of Education. Dental treatment for schoolchildren became compulsory in England after the Education Act of 1921, meals for primary[28] school children were provided from 1904 and free school milk from 1934.

Attention in this period also began to be paid to working conditions. Safety at work and occupational health became an important part of public health from 1910 in many countries, including the UK, with health and sanitary inspection of workplaces.

III) NUTRITION AND FLUORIDATION

The science of nutrition developed at the start of the twentieth century to prevent and tackle dietary deficiency and understand the health benefits of different foods, vitamins and minerals. In the United States, for example, the Pure Food and Drugs Act of 1906 established food and labelling standards. In 1911, the chemical nature of vitamin D was identified and the incidence of rickets declined following its fortification in milk.

Before the introduction of fluoridated toothpaste in the 1970s, there were existing schemes to add fluoride to drinking water to prevent tooth decay. The US had pilot schemes from 1945 and the Department of Health in the UK promoted fluoridation from 1955. Despite strong evidence of effectiveness and safety, this remains a contentious issue, however, and has not been universally implemented in any of the 40 countries with fluoridation schemes in place.

IV) THE PROFESSIONALISATION OF THE PUBLIC HEALTH WORKFORCE

The turn of the century also saw a continued growth in professional public health organisations. In 1910, the Canadian Public Health Association was created by a small group of physicians concerned about the state of public health. In France, the first national organisations dealing with public health, the Société Française d'Hygiène and La Société de Médicine Publique et d'Hygiène Professionnelle, were accorded state approval in 1900. In England, the Association of Medical Officers of Health, launched in 1856 became the Society of Medical Officers of Health in 1908 and, after mergers and changes in name, became the current Royal Society for Public

Health in 2008.[29] From 1886 its members needed to have a public health qualification. The Association of Directors of Public Health was established in 1989. In Germany, the National Society for Public Health had been founded in 1873 and the Prussian Medical Officers Law of 1899 provided full time Medical Officers of Health within State employment.

In the USA, there was a battle between physicians, on the one hand, and scientists and technicians on the other hand, for dominance of public health. While doctors still retained a privileged status, schools of public health took in nurses, engineers, statisticians and biologists. The first multidisciplinary school was opened in 1916 at John Hopkins University with a grant from the Rockefeller Foundation which later supported other schools.[30]

There was increasingly recognition that central organisation was needed to achieve public health objectives rather than relying on the efforts of a combination of local authorities and voluntary associations. In 1900, the first public health department under ministerial control was established in New Zealand. In Canada, following the start of the Spanish flu pandemic in 1918, the Federal Department of Health was founded in 1919 as was the Ministry of Health in Britain.

V) THE RISE OF SOCIAL MEDICINE AND EUGENICS

Following this work on disease prevention in populations, a new theory emerged after the First World War. This looked at the relationship between medicine and social factors and aimed to blend preventive and curative approaches. This rise in 'social medicine' was influenced by developments in Russia. After the October Revolution in 1917, social hygiene departments were established, based on the recognition that improvement in mainly material conditions (now described as social determinants) would result in lower disease and death rates. The Russian state health plan of 1918 created a comprehensive health system, with emphasis on prevention, which covered maternal and child health care as well as responses to epidemics and communicable disease control. All services were provided free through a network of polyclinics, maternity clinics and child-care centres.

Eugenics (meaning 'good breeding') or the science – now discredited – of increasing the occurrence of heritable characteristics regarded as desirable in the population, was an unpleasant and unintended side effect of social medicine. It influenced people in several countries, including the UK and USA, to view those with poorer health, or other unpopular characteristics, as inferior. In the UK, at one point, there was a campaign for voluntary sterilisation targeted at those considered to have hereditary 'defects'. In the Germany of the Weimar Republic in the 1920s, eugenics offered a rationale for medical control over a vast range of welfare services. It later led to the Nazi concept of a 'master race' when medical officers were given an increasingly important role in implementing highly discriminatory and ultimately lethal racial and population policies. In Sweden, there was the desire to improve the general health of the working population in the belief that bad habits had to be rectified. The largely rural country at the time could not support the population expansion that had occurred. Between the end of the nineteenth and early twentieth centuries, about 1.3 million people, or 20 per cent of the population, left the country, mainly for the United States. In the United States, there were concerns about the deterioration of national 'stock' and the idea that biologically inferior immigrants were responsible for the growing statistics of physical disease, alcohol dependence, mental illness, urban violence and criminality.

The early decades of the twentieth century saw, therefore, a complete shift in public health focus, driven by the poor state of health of populations and fuelled by new – and sometimes dangerous – ideas on prevention.

4. A FOCUS ON HEALTH CARE AND THE DEVELOPMENT OF WELFARE STATES

The first two decades of the twentieth century had seen a burgeoning of programmes to tackle maternal and child health issues – such as malnutrition, vison and hearing problems, poor dental health – whilst also expanding services to combat infectious diseases. From the 1930s, however, the emphasis of governments shifted away from public health measures to the contribution made by health services to better health. In the UK, the public health service was to become largely the province of local government responsible for sanitation services and food safety as well as a raft of welfare services for mothers and children, clinics for TB and running the former Poor Law hospitals.[31]

The discovery of penicillin[32] in 1928 introduced a new era of antibiotics and an increasingly technological approach to disease management. The British government's focus was on the provision of health services for the bulk of the population. With the Great Depression of the 1930s and then the rebuilding of societies needed after the Second World, the focus shifted to setting up the welfare state. Internationally, different models and funding mechanisms for the provision of health and social care were established.

I) HEALTH SYSTEM IN THE UK

The 1911 National Insurance Act introduced by the Prime Minister at the time, Lloyd George, provided compulsory health insurance for workers. The health system until the Second World War was, however, confused, split between private General Practitioner (GP) services, local authority public health departments led by the MOH[33] and charitable voluntary hospitals staffed by consultants. The National Health Service (NHS), established in 1948, without the support of the British Medical Association (BMA)[34] until the last moment, provided a universal system with healthcare free at the point of use, funded not primarily by insurance, but by general taxation. The new system nevertheless retained the previous tripartite system (separate hospital, primary care and public health systems), with public health and community services located in local government, GPs remaining as independent contractors to the health service and consultants deployed in state-owned hospitals. The focus of the NHS was more on treatment and cure rather than prevention.

MOsH, with the loss of much of their 'empire', when control of all hospitals moved to the new health service in 1948, were still responsible for public health, delivering community health services and environmental health departments. It was not until the 1974 health services' reorganisation that public health doctors were moved out of local government and into the NHS along with community health provision (but not environmental health which has always remained a local government function).[35] From this time, coinciding with the creation of the Faculty of Public Health (FPH)[36] in 1972, specialist public health doctors achieved equivalence to medical consultants in the NHS and began to have somewhat more influence within the healthcare system.

II) HEALTH SYSTEMS IN EUROPE

In the 1920s, national health insurance schemes developed in many countries in Europe, based on a system established in 1883 in Germany by Otto von Bismarck. He introduced compulsory national health insurance to ensure healthy workers and army recruits. Following this, the Weimar welfare state saw a large-scale building programme of hospitals and health centres.

In France, where two thirds of French communes in the 1930s still lacked adequate supplies of safe drinking water, it was not until after the Second World War that improvements in public health took place along with the construction of an extensive healthcare system. A medical social insurance law was introduced in 1930 which was compulsory for industrial and commercial employees whose earnings were below a certain level. Patients paid the physician directly, then would be reimbursed up to 80% of the costs. The system was independent of State bureaucracy. Following the Second World War, the scheme expanded into a comprehensive social security system for the whole population, covering not only sickness but also welfare benefits to families, old age pensions and disability.

In Sweden, the miseries of the 1930s Depression led to the building of the modern welfare state. Measures were taken to reform medical care, child-care and maternity care.[37] This national project was based on the principle of equal access to health care and prevention services as an individual right. Services were provided at little or no cost to the individual by public institutions and delivered by publicly funded professionals through a network of health centres.

Italy, like Britain, established a tax funded national health service in 1978. This guaranteed provision of comprehensive health services to the whole population. Public health in Italy was not seen as separate from the publicly funded health care services, however. Responsibility for health services was shared between central government and 21 regions and autonomous provinces, with central government providing the legislative framework. There was no overarching public health act or central public health agency.

III) HEALTH SYSTEMS IN FRONTIER COUNTRIES

In Canada, national pensions and national health insurance programmes were developed after the Second World War. Government health insurance had been discussed in the 1930s but had led to a doctors' strike and been abandoned. Legislation in 1957 set up an agreement between the Federal Government and Provinces to establish a comprehensive insurance plan covering acute hospital care, laboratory and diagnostic services. Immunisation programmes were established from the 1950s, but doctors continued to remain wary of State medicine.

There was a similar story in Australia and New Zealand where doctors continued to resist state encroachment. In New Zealand, doctors thwarted government attempts in 1935 to introduce free health care to hospitals and to GPs. In Australia, opposition from the medical profession led to the abandonment of the Federal Government's National Health and Pensions Insurance Act of 1939. Doctors then rejected the setting up of a national health service in 1948 for fear of nationalisation. A national health service was eventually introduced in 1949 on a fee-for-service basis, financed by government, supported by a subsidised insurance programme. In both countries the health of indigenous people continued to be a largely neglected public health challenge.

In the United States, there was no recognisable welfare state until the Great Depression, when the 1935 Federal Social Security Act expanded the financing of the public health service. It also provided federal grants to States to help them develop public health services with programmes to control specific diseases. There continued to be opposition to what was perceived as 'socialised medicine' so that partial universal coverage – for the over 65s (Medicare) and 'the poor' (Medicaid) – was not introduced until 1965. Private health insurance is still the main method of funding US health care. Public health agencies were, and still are, seen largely as social agencies directed to the needs of people on lowest incomes and minority populations.

5. THE IMPACT OF MODERN ENVIRONMENTS AND BEHAVIOURS ON HEALTH AND A RENEWED EMPHASIS ON COMMUNICABLE DISEASES

From the end of the Second World War in 1945, policy had shifted to cure and treatment with increasing involvement of states in medicine and social welfare through hospital provision and primary care (GP) services. Alongside advances in medicine and technological aspects of care came the extension of social medicine ideas that good health was linked to factors such as occupation, education, food and income. Medical science was not going to be the only answer to health problems, however. John Ryle, Britain's first professor of social medicine, considered that man must be treated 'as a whole'.[38]

I) A MORE HOLISTIC APPROACH TO HEALTH AND PREVENTION

As average life expectancy and the general health of Western populations rose following the institution of welfare states, the public health focus shifted once more. This time it was to health problems stemming from the modern environment such as tobacco, alcohol, drugs, diet, physical inactivity and, latterly, climate change. Cardiovascular disease was an early cause of concern and, more recently, rising levels of obesity accompanied by metabolic and other serious disorders. Lobbying for government action on these issues became a key public health activity.

Health care demands and costs were also rising in the face of both increasing and ageing populations, chronic disease and the need to fund medical advances. An early response came from Canada. In his 1974 report, *A New Perspective on the Health of Canadians*,[39] Marc Lalonde, the Canadian Minister of National Health and Welfare, rejected the dominance of the prevailing medical model of health and advocated a more holistic understanding of health and a broader approach to public health. He asserted that this was through healthy living and an appreciation of the breadth of factors that determine health. He identified four major components in his Health Field Concept – human biology (genetics), health care systems, environment, and lifestyle.

The report shifted government priorities from treatment to prevention with a focus on risk factors to health – the so-called 'new' public health. There were health promotion campaigns, and efforts to reduce harms to health such as from smoking, traffic accidents and alcohol abuse. Lalonde's report was followed internationally by the World Health Organization's (WHO) Declaration of Alma Ata in 1978,[40] which expressed the need for urgent action by all governments, health and development workers and the world community to protect and promote the health of all people. Broader health promotion goals, and an understanding of social and economic determinants of health, led to a new movement to address the links between poverty and ill-health. This approach was emphasised in the international Ottawa Charter for Health Promotion in 1986.

II) THE EMERGENCE OF HEALTH INEQUALITIES AS AN ISSUE

Health inequalities emerged as an important issue in the 1970s, particularly in Britain. It has long been recognised that some people live to a healthy old age while others succumb to a variety of diseases earlier in life or die prematurely. Over the past half century considerable research has taken place into the causes of these differences, establishing they were the result of a range of determinants of health and ill-health.[41] Since the Black Report[42] on inequalities and health was published in 1980, it has been widely known that people's social circumstances – such as living in less affluent areas, having low incomes and lower educational attainment – affect their health experience negatively. Commissioned by an outgoing Labour Government, the working group was chaired by Sir Douglas Black, then England's Chief Medical Officer, who was a Scottish physician and medical scientist. The report was received by the incoming Conservative Government of Margaret Thatcher who found the recommendations unpalatable – to the extent of replacing publicly the term 'inequalities' with 'variations' in health, with the implication that these differences between population groups could be due to chance – resulting in minimal government action.[43] The report did show beyond doubt, however, that ill health and death were distributed unequally among the population of Britain. Moreover, inequalities had widened rather than decreased since the start of the NHS in 1948. This confirmed earlier work from the Whitehall Study of British civil servants, initially begun in 1967 and led by Sir Michael Marmot (Professor of Epidemiology at University College London), which showed a steep inverse association among civil servants between social class and deaths from a wide range of diseases.

It was not until the Labour Government of Tony Blair, elected in 1997, that further work was commissioned in England on health inequalities and a commitment made to address them. This work was led initially by Sir Donald Acheson, then England's Chief Medical Officer, and Sir Michael Marmot. Recommendations to address inequalities were published and initially some policies were introduced, for example the Sure Start programme to support families with children under 5, targeted at the poorest areas. The actions of successive governments since these reports have made little impact overall, however, and in recent years the gap has widened between those living the most healthy lives and those the least.[44] Indeed, health inequalities in Britain also worsened during the COVID-19 pandemic as employment and financial insecurity, as well as the virus itself, affected different sectors of society disproportionately.[45,46] This will be discussed further in Chapter 7.

III) NEW AND RE-EMERGING COMMUNICABLE DISEASES

This most recent era has also seen communicable diseases return as a major public health issue. The emergence of new infections, notably the AIDS epidemic from the early 1980s, sent shock waves round the world and returned public health efforts to the fore in the prevention and management of blood-borne and sexually transmitted diseases. Since then, other infectious diseases have emerged or re-emerged – including poliomyelitis (polio), measles, Ebola, Severe Acue Respiratory Syndrome (SARS), Middle East Respiratory Syndrome (MERS), COVID-19 and Mpox. Some of the spread derives from increased global travel. Some is due to poor vaccine uptake. There is constant watch for the next influenza pandemic. Malaria has remained a prominent threat and scourge, mainly in low-income countries largely neglected by the wealthy northern nations. We shall return to this in Chapter 10.

6. RECENT INITIATIVES TO IMPROVE THE MANAGEMENT OF HEALTH AND DISEASE

I) SCREENING PROGRAMMES

During the latter third of the twentieth century national programmes were introduced for preventing ill health through screening, spearheaded by public health action, and compliant with the evidence base, to determine, for the nation, the most appropriate and affordable eligibility such as age group/s, gender (where applicable) and frequency of screening. The NHS defines screening as a way of systematically identifying at an early stage, apparently healthy people who are susceptible to developing a serious medical condition, most often a type of cancer.[47] Breast cancer screening was introduced in the NHS for women aged 50 and over following the publication of the Forrest Report in 1986. Screening for cervical cancer was in place in the UK in an uncoordinated way from the 1960s, with the formal NHS programme beginning in 1988, for women[48] between 25 and 65 years of age.

For men, the NHS national abdominal aortic aneurism screening programme was introduced in 2008. For everyone over the age of 60 years, bowel cancer screening has been offered since 2006.

Since 2008, the cervical screening programme has been complemented by the national HPV (Human papillomavirus) vaccination programme for school children, which provides protection against cervical and some other cancers. Combatting cervical cancer has been an important public health success story of the modern era. In time, when most adults are protected by the vaccine, this screening programme, which has saved thousands of lives, may no longer be needed.

II) EVIDENCE-BASED MEDICINE

A major public health tool developed from the 1970s onwards is evidence-based medicine. This aimed to make clinical medicine and the health services safer and more effective by a focus on what clinical management is known to be effective and ceasing procedures and treatments for which there was no, or insufficient, evidence of benefit. The seminal work on this subject, *Effectiveness and Efficiency: Random Reflections on Health Services*, published in 1972,[49] was written by Archie Cochrane, a Scottish physician, epidemiologist and medical researcher.

III) RANDOMISED CONTROLLED TRIALS AND ACCESSING PATIENTS' VIEWS ON HEALTH CARE

Cochrane pioneered the use of randomised controlled trials (RCTs) as the 'gold standard' for clinical research. Examples of evidence-based practice included recognition that routinely removing tonsils, or inserting grommets, for example, were not necessarily in children's best interests. A more selective, evidence-based and efficient allocation of limited resources was needed, to ensure that surgery was performed only on the children who were most likely to benefit.

In addition to objective evidence from research, particularly from RCTs, more subjective evidence began to be recognised for its value in service improvement, including, importantly, the role of patients' views. Patient representatives were introduced into decision-making in health care in the UK to take into account of acceptability and understanding of services. There was later development by public health researchers of tools such as patient reported outcome measures (PROMS), to help balance the reliance on professional, technical or financial views of effectiveness.

IV) MODERNISING THE PUBLIC HEALTH WORKFORCE

The expertise to tackle public health issues also evolved during this period, to reflect the differing demands and approaches needed. Whereas previously the more senior public health workforce had been led by those with medical qualifications, in England and Wales there was formal recognition from 2002[50] of the contribution made to public health by senior personnel from a variety of backgrounds and expertise – health promotion, health intelligence, health services and generalists – to the extent that the specialist workforce has been multidisciplinary at senior level since 2002.[51]

In some countries, the public health workforce remains primarily medically led as in France, and also in Italy where it forms part of the healthcare service.[52] In the United States, from early days as we have seen, the workforce has been multidisciplinary.

NOTES

1 Popularised by Charles Townshend in the eighteenth century, the Norfolk crop rotation meant land was used intensively by planting wheat, turnips, barley and clover on a four-year cycle avoiding a fallow year.
2 The causes of this mortality decline are debated by historians. The decline is probably due to several factors including better personal hygiene, the natural decline in diseases such as smallpox and better nutrition.
3 https://www.victorianlondon.org/population/population.htm
4 https://www.hslc.org.uk/wp-content/uploads/2017/05/122-5-Taylor.pdf

5 A humanitarian is a person promoting human welfare and social reform. Nineteenth-century English humanitarians were involved in a wide range of causes, including prison reform, public health, and the abolition of slavery.

6 Mortality and morbidity will be explained more fully later, but for now read 'death' and 'ill health', respectively.

7 The first British Census was in 1801 but 1841 is usually regarded as the first modern Census.

8 Farr had studied in Paris under Pierre Charles Alexandre Louis, responsible for developing the 'méthode numérique'. Louis divided patients into exposed/affected versus unexposed/unaffected groups in order to determine the relationship between illness and its causes. He conducted several observational studies including one that showed bloodletting was ineffective. His method was a precursor of epidemiology.

9 The 1834 Poor Law ensured that destitute families could be housed in workhouses and receive food and clothing in return for work.

10 Miasma is the Ancient Greek word for pollution.

11 These Acts would not apply, of course, to those doing piece work in their own homes.

12 A national government is a single, central government authority. A federal government is one that splits power with its 'units' (like states).

13 APHA. https://www.apha.org/getcontentasset/b8e5b607-5b0a-40fb-8f44-72b9767c05b6/7ca0dc9d-611d-46e2-9fd3-26a4c03ddcbb/apha2022_history_installation.pdf?language=en

14 McCready was a physician who worked on the cholera and typhus epidemics; Shattuck was called the architect of American public health who promoted the keeping of accurate health statistics; Griscom, a chemist, founded New York's anti-poverty programme.

15 Specific areas of land designation for Native American tribes.

16 In 1904 the Department of the Interior and of Indian Affairs in Canada appointed a medical officer to organise and supervise the health of indigenous populations.

17 The passing of a disease from one individual to another by direct or indirect contact.

18 Microbes are tiny living organisms, too small to be seen by the naked eye, that live in water, soil and air as well as on and inside humans and other living creatures.

19 Anton van Leeuwenhoek, an early eighteenth-century Dutch scientist, was the first to see and describe bacteria through a microscope.

20 A type of bacterium.
21 Organisms, such as biting insects or ticks that transmits a disease from one creature to another.
22 Aseptic is the absence of infection.
23 The process of preventing the growth of infectious germs, like bacteria, viruses and fungi.
24 From the Latin for cow (*vacca*), because of the early use of the cowpox virus against smallpox.
25 The law has recently been extended to include chickenpox.
26 Postnatal care is care given to newborns and their parents in the critical period following birth.
27 Holding a nursing qualification first before training as a health visitor only became a requirement from 1945.
28 Called 'elementary schools' in this period; for children aged 5–11 years.
29 Its journal, *Public Health*, has been in continuous publication since 1888.
30 Multidisciplinary schools of public health did not appear in the UK until the late 1990s at Cardiff.
31 The Poor Law was a framework, dating from the sixteenth century, for local parishes to raise taxes to support those unable to work.
32 By Alexander Fleming in 1928; further research by Florey and Chain meant that penicillin became available for medical use during the Second World War, then available for public use in the UK from 1946.
33 Responsible for environmental health, maternity and child welfare clinics, health visiting, family planning, and, from 1928, management of the former Poor Law hospitals.
34 The trade union representing doctors and medical students.
35 The 2013 reorganisation of the health service in England moved Directors of Public Health and their teams back into local government along with a specific public health budget to cover functions such as health improvement programmes, smoking cessation, substance misuse services, etc.
36 Originally called the Faculty of Community Medicine, now the Faculty of Public Health of the Royal Colleges of Physicians.
37 As well as property rents, the pensions system, higher education.
38 https://pmc.ncbi.nlm.nih.gov/articles/PMC10482575/
39 https://nccdh.ca/resources/entry/new-perspective-on-the-health-of-canadians
40 https://www.globalfamilydoctor.com/site/DefaultSite/filesystem/documents/starfield/declaration_almaata.pdf

41 See Dahlgren and Whitehead in the Introduction, p. 4.

42 Black, D., Morris, J., Smith, C. and Townshend, P. *Inequalities in Health: Report of a Research Working Group* (also known as the 'Black Report') DHSS, 30 August 1980.

43 A subsequent Labour Government did publish a cross-government Action Plan in 2003 (23 years after publication of the Black Report).

44 See his initial report: Marmot, M. *Fair Society, Healthy Lives – Strategic Review of Health Inequalities*, London: Institute of Health Equity, 2010.

45 https://www.health.org.uk/reports-and-analysis/briefings/the-continuing-impact-of-covid-19-on-health-and-inequalities

46 https://www.bma.org.uk/advice-and-support/covid-19/what-the-bma-is-doing/the-impact-of-the-pandemic-on-population-health-and-health-inequalities

47 https://www.nhs.uk/tests-and-treatments/nhs-screening/

48 Biological females with a cervix.

49 https://www.nuffieldtrust.org.uk/sites/default/files/2017-01/effectiveness-and-efficiency-web-final.pdf

50 Scotland and Northern Ireland were slower to adopt multidisciplinary health at the specialist level.

51 This was after a long battle for recognition by those in public health at a senior level but not medically trained. For the full history see Wright, J., Sim. F. and Ferguson, K. *Multidisciplinary Public Health: Understanding the Development of the Modern Workforce*, Policy Press, 2016

52 https://www.ncbi.nlm.nih.gov/books/NBK507328/; https://www.ncbi.nlm.nih.gov/books/NBK535727/

2

PUBLIC HEALTH IN LOW- AND MIDDLE-INCOME COUNTRIES

1. COLONIALISM

Public health in countries beyond the Western World had varied trajectories following the different histories of these countries and, for many, their colonial past. Colonialism (which has been defined as 'control by one power over a dependent area or people')[1] by western countries meant that full industrialisation and modernisation did not occur, for the most part, until at least the middle of the twentieth century, coinciding with the end of the imperial era, as countries moved from colonial to more democratised public health systems.

Colonial control was epitomised by economic exploitation and control of trade, land and labour with little incentive to invest in the country's health and welfare, even in times of epidemics and famine. The examples detailed below relate to circumstances in India and sub-Saharan Africa. A similar tale could be told, however, for western management of the Middle East, South America and for Japan's control of its colonies in the Far East.[2]

In India and Africa, initial public health measures were typically only for colonists and those who worked for them and in urban centres rather than rural communities, creating inequalities. There was also opposition from local populations against imposed health regimes which were contrary to their religions and cultures, and established trusted local health and medical practices. There was a misfit between the colonial-derived model and the needs of the mass of the population. Therefore, imposition of a western model of sanitation and medicine did not work well.

DOI: 10.4324/9781003779902-4

2. COLONIALISM IN INDIA

Colonialism in India was different from Africa in that the British East India Company had been an important presence there from the seventeenth century. By the middle of the eighteenth had established areas it ruled, which it continued to expand until the Government of India Act of 1858 led to the British controlling present-day Bangladesh, Pakistan and India. Following an adverse report in 1863 on the sanitary conditions of the army, in 1869 a Public Health Commissioner and Statistical Officer were appointed to the Government of India, with representation in each province responsible for public health matters – including surveys, planning and regulation.

Communicable diseases regularly ravaging the region included plague, leprosy, cholera and malaria. Whilst brutal methods were used to control epidemics – forceful segregation of infected persons, disinfection, evacuation and sometimes demolition of infected places, the government also undertook research into the diseases to understand how they were transmitted and how they could then be controlled. By the first half of the twentieth century, mortality from epidemics had fallen and the British Imperial Government set up an organised medical system. Progress was slow because of a combination of factors including lack of funds and hostility from the local population. Following India's independence in 1947 its First Five Year Plan noted that only 3% of households had toilets and most of the population lacked water, drainage and waste disposal services.

3. COLONIALISM IN AFRICA

Colonialism came to Africa towards the end of the nineteenth century. The Berlin conference of 1884/5, known as the 'Scramble for Africa',[3] effectively divided the continent among European powers (Britain, France, Germany, Portugal, Belgium, Italy and Spain). The colonial medical and public health services mirrored those in Europe, in the belief that a simple transfer of their ideology and technology would address what they saw as widespread ignorance, lack of sanitation and poor health. As in India, the earliest medical efforts of colonialists were to protect the health of Europeans and indigenous populations in their service, as exposure to new diseases took their toll on the colonialist European populations. Outbreaks of sleeping sickness in the early 1900s, spread by the tsetse fly and lethal before the era of modern treatments, were an important factor in encouraging the colonials to take a broader approach to public health problems and to start annual public health surveys.

The interwar years saw rapid urbanisation and slum development, as the need for labour in towns increased, but there were no coherent public health programmes. There was resistance from Africans to the imposition of western customs of hygiene. Rural family lives were often disrupted as men left to work in urban areas on a seasonal basis. This labour mobility led to widespread transmission among rural communities of diseases such as syphilis, more usually associated with urban life.

4. THE LEGACY OF COLONIALISM IN LMICS

Most colonies in Africa did not achieve independence until the 1960s.The focus from the international community in the immediate post-war period was on building hospitals and importing western diagnostic and therapeutic technology. After independence, low- and middle-income countries (LMICs) suffered from lack of effective preventive and control measures for smallpox, plague, yellow fever and cholera. Limited resources and overspending on high-tech hospital facilities in large cities also left inadequate funding for developing affordable primary care services for both rural and urban communities.

In the 1970s, there was an emerging appreciation that focusing on highly expensive hospital care was not necessarily most appropriate to meet the health needs of these populations. Developing primary health care became seen as a cheaper solution, alongside public health measures – chiefly vaccination and provision of clean water – in tackling the underlying causes of disease and ill-health. The 1978 WHO declaration of Alma Ata focused on primary health care, promoting healthy food and nutrition, safe water and basic sanitation. It advocated public health education campaigns on health problems and their prevention, maternal and child health including family planning (sexual health, contraception), and vaccination and immunisation.

Collective efforts in more recent years, therefore, have been in part to rectify the legacy of colonial approaches and institutions and develop bottom-up approaches in partnership with local communities, rather than externally imposed solutions. These aim to define services which are country appropriate and to empower LMICs to recognise and celebrate their own assets as well as supporting them to address their population health challenges.

Cholera is still a significant global public health problem, as is plague, and yellow fever is endemic in many LMICs. Malaria remains a huge cause of death particularly among children, with vaccines only recently being developed. AIDS remains a global problem with the highest burden in the twenty-first century borne by Sub-Saharan Africa and Southeast Asia. Access to effective preventive measures for malaria and drugs for HIV infection have been limited in comparison to higher income countries, with insufficient priority given to international efforts to tackle these inequities. Alongside communicable diseases in recent decades, LMICs have experienced increasing problems previously associated with western lifestyles, with incidence of cardiovascular disease, obesity, diabetes and some cancers all increasing. In recent decades the people in many LMICs have also been subject to famine, terrorism and war.

NOTES

1 https://www.nationalgeographic.com/culture/article/colonialism#:~:text=Merriam%2DWebster%20defines%20colonialism%20as,and%20culture%20on%20the%20locals

2 For discussion on these legacies see Liu, M.S., 'From Colonial Medicine to International Health in East Asia', https://humanitiesfutures.org/papers/from-colonial-medicine-to-international-health-in-east-asia/; Asi, Y.M., 'The Colonial Legacy in the Arab World: Health, Education and Politics', 9 November 2022, https://arabcenterdc.org/resource/the-colonial-legacy-in-the-arab-world-health-education-and-politics/; Cueto, M. and Palmer, S., 'History of Public Health in Latin America', 25 February 2017, https://oxfordre.com/publichealth/display/10.1093/acrefore/9780190632366.001.0001/acrefore-9780190632366-e-20?d=%2F10.1093%2Facrefore%2F9780190632366.001.0001%2Facrefore-9780190632366

3 Britannica.com/event/scramble-for-Africa

3

INTERNATIONAL AND GLOBAL APPROACHES TO PUBLIC HEALTH

Collective effort to improve public health has been in existence since the nineteenth century with an acknowledgement of the need for countries to work together at an international level. This has not only been seen in delivering aid to LMICs, but in surveillance systems and responses to continuing and emerging communicable and non-communicable diseases.

The debate continues, however, over the scope of global public health, whether it should be narrow and focus on health threats across countries or whether it should also address social, economic and political determinants of health and equity, and whether it should it be reactive or proactive?[1]

There have been limits in practice on the extent of international cooperation and governance as we shall see in Part 3 when we look at specific health challenges.

1. INITIAL COLLABORATIONS

The first international sanitary conference on health statistics took place in 1853. It established the basis for an agreed classification of the causes of death. It was followed by other international conferences on a range of topics relating to specific health issues. Attendees comprised a mix of government representatives, charities and local professionals. Many of these conferences led to the setting up of international campaigns, for example against TB.

In 1907, the first international organisation, the International Office of Public Health, was established. Its function was to gather and distribute epidemiological information on infectious diseases.

DOI: 10.4324/9781003779902-5

After the First World War, in 1923 the League of Nations set up a Health Organization (LNHO). Initially, it focused on additional international standard setting of health statistics but during the Depression in the 1930s it worked with the League of Nations International Labour Office (ILO) to look at the impact of diet, housing and economic conditions on human health. It was also the first attempt to create effective programmes on a large scale for tackling disease starting with malaria and moving on to TB, syphilis, rabies, leprosy, cancer and sleeping sickness. Some of these activities were carried out with the help of the Rockefeller Foundation in the United States which, in 1913, had founded an International Health Division. This supported research, training of personnel and funds on a temporary basis to set up community health services in LMICs which, at that time, were identified as developing countries.

2. THE ESTABLISHMENT AND WORK OF THE WORLD HEALTH ORGANIZATION

Collaborative international initiatives provided the basis for further joint work after the Second World War. The LNHO merged with the post-war United National Relief and Rehabilitation Administration (UNRAA) and the Office of International Hygiene to form the World Health Organization (WHO) in 1948. The WHO also absorbed tasks from the International Office of Public Health. Under the umbrella of the United Nations, the WHO has become the official worldwide coordinating agency in international health. The WHO's global headquarters are in Geneva. It operates through six Regional Offices and offices in 150 countries.[2] The WHO provides technical assistance to countries, sets international health standards, collects data on global health issues, and serves as a forum for scientific or policy discussions related to health. It played a leading role in the eradication of smallpox.[3] It is governed by the World Health Assembly and is funded by contributions from its 194 member states.[4] In 1981, WHO followed the Alma Ata conference with the ambitious 'Health for All by the Year 2000' target.[5] This emphasised the importance of intersectoral working towards improved public health involving housing, transport and education.

3. UNITED NATIONS INITIATIVES

Until the discovery of effective drugs, the main means to combat HIV/AIDS was to urge individuals to be aware of how it spread and to educate them about safer sex and provide the means to protect themselves. Crucial also was the need to ensure the safety of blood products. The Joint United Nations Programme on HIV and AIDS (UNAIDS) was set up in 1994. Its function was to coordinate the global response to the disease and provide technical support.

A further joint programme, Roll Back Malaria (RBM), was launched in 1998 to coordinate a global response.[6]

4. SHARED SURVEILLANCE

Emphasis has also been placed globally on improved disease surveillance through sharing of intelligence data. This is important in controlling the spread of communicable disease. In most countries routine surveillance data are sent to national agencies which then analyse and distribute information on disease trends at regional or global level. These agencies also receive data from countries when the impact of a public health event crosses borders. This is to help prevent threats that have the potential to affect populations worldwide. One example of this is the Global Influenza Surveillance and Response System, a laboratory network that shares information to detect the emergence of novel (newly discovered) influenza viruses with pandemic potential. This helped prevent SARS[7] from becoming endemic in many countries after the 2002–4 pandemic. Public health data are not always shared freely, however, because of perceived or real technical, political, economic or legal barriers. This was apparent in the MERS[8] outbreak that commenced in 2012, when reluctance to share data delayed assessment of the disease origin. Subsequent disease outbreaks caused by the Ebola virus from 2014, and Zika virus from 2016, then COVID-19 since 2019, have increased awareness of the importance of data sharing among health stakeholders internationally, though challenges remain.

Important national and international intelligence agencies include the United States Centers for Disease Prevention and Control (CDC). This is a federal agency which acts to detect and respond to new and emerging health threats in addition to its overarching disease surveillance and control functions.[9] Another is the European Centre for Disease Prevention and Control (ECDC) which was established in 2005. Its aim is to strengthen Europe's defence against infectious diseases by collecting, collating, evaluating and disseminating relevant scientific and technical data. The Africa Centres for Disease Control and Prevention were formed in 2016. The UK Health Security Agency (UKHSA),[10] developed from its predecessor Public Health England (during the COVID-19 pandemic) and prior to that the UK Health Protection Agency, is the government agency, sponsored by the Department of Health and Social Care which prevents, prepares for, and responds to, communicable disease, environmental and chemical hazards working with local, national and international organisations.

5. OTHER ORGANISATIONS WORKING FOR INTERNATIONAL HEALTH

Other major organisations involved in global health include the World Bank and the Gates Foundation for world-wide research and project delivery. The World Bank is one of the largest financial contributors to health-related projects. In 1979, it set up a division for direct lending for health, which helps countries to develop primary health systems and provide quality, affordable health services to everyone regardless of their ability to pay. It also operates as a 'knowledge bank' providing expertise to countries on health policy and financing.

The Gates Foundation was established by Bill and Melinda Gates in 2000 for work covering HIV/AIDS, TB, malaria and immunisation. It is the largest charitable foundation in the United States. Its stated goal is to reduce inequities and improve lives round the world. Since 2000, it has made available over 79 billion dollars and is also one of the top financial contributors to the WHO.

In addition to data sharing, there are organisations which send teams to assist in health emergencies wherever they occur in the world. CDC, for example, has 400 experts ready to respond to a public health emergency anywhere in the world within 72 hours of the declared emergency.

International health is the focus of the European Health Observatory, established in 1998 and hosted by the WHO Europe. The Observatory supports development of the evidence base, which, by effective communication with policy makers, supports them in running, reforming and strengthening health systems throughout the WHO European Region.

6. A COMMON FRAMEWORK FOR DELIVERING PUBLIC HEALTH FUNCTIONS

As we have seen, each country differs in its structure of public health systems and workforce. There is now some agreement, however, on what all should include as essential public health services. This builds on the historical development of public health and what is needed now to respond to global issues. The first list of Essential Public Health Functions was published in 1998 by the WHO and updated in 2023 as follows:[11]

- **Public health surveillance and monitoring**: monitoring and surveillance of population health status, risk, protective and promotive factors, threats to health, and health system performance and service use.
- **Public health emergency management**: managing public health emergencies.
- **Public health stewardship**: establishing effective public health institutional structures, leadership, coordination, accountability, and regulations and legislations.
- **Multisectoral planning and financing for public health**: supporting effective and efficient health systems and multisectoral planning, financing and management for public health.
- **Health protection**: protecting populations against health threats, including environment and occupational hazards, communicable and non-communicable diseases including mental health conditions, food insecurity, chemical and radiation hazards.
- **Disease prevention**: prevention and early detection of communicable and non-communicable diseases including mental health conditions, and injuries.
- **Health promotion**: promoting health and well-being as well as actions to address the wider determinants of health and inequity.
- **Community engagement and social participation**: strengthening community engagement, participation and social mobilisation for health and well-being.
- **Public health workforce development**: developing and maintaining an adequate and competent public health workforce.

- **Health service quality and equity**: improving the appropriateness, quality, equity in provision and access of health services.
- **Public health research and knowledge**: advancing public health research and knowledge development.
- **Access to and use of health products, supplies, equipment and technologies**: promoting the equitable access to and rational use of safe, effective and quality assured health products, supplies, equipment and technologies.

These features of a modern public health system will be explored further in Part 2 when we look at terminology, public health competence and the workforces needed to deliver public health services.

NOTES

1 Galea, S. and Annas, G., 'An Argument for a Common-sense Global Public Health Agenda', *The Lancet Public Health*, October 2017, 2(10). https://www.thelancet.com/journals/lanpub/article/PIIS2468-2667(17)30164-0/fulltext
2 https://www.who.int/about/structure
3 Through its Smallpox Eradication Programme, launched in 1959, to coordinate international effort. https://www.who.int/news-room/spotlight/history-of-vaccination/history-of-smallpox-vaccination
4 Several other agencies under the United Nations umbrella emerged to help deal with health, social and economic development such as the UN Development Programme (UNDP), the UN Children's Fund (UNICEF), the UN Population Fund (UNFPA) the UN High Commissioner for Refugees (UNHCR), UN AIDS.
5 https://digitallibrary.un.org/record/32711?ln=en
6 https://apps.who.int/gb/ebwha/pdf_files/WHA52/ew6.pdf; https://data.unaids.org/pub/report/2008/jc1579_first_10_years_en.pdf
7 SARS (Severe Acute Respiratory Syndrome) was first identified in China in 2002. It went on to infect over 8,000 people in 30 countries.
8 MERS (Middle East Respiratory Syndrome) outbreak was first identified in Saudi Arabia in 2012 and spread to several countries, mainly in the Middle East.
9 Threatened by cuts by the current US administration.
10 Previously the Health Protection Agency before Public Health England.
11 Squires, N., Garfield, R., Mohammed-Ahmed, O., Iversen, B.G., Tegnell, A. et al., 'Essential Public Health Functions: The Key to Resilient Health Systems', *BMJ Global Health* 12 July 2023, Editorial. https://gh.bmj.com/content/8/7/e013136

SUMMARY

'Modern' public health includes a mixture of state, regional and locally funded and delivered services. It is an amalgam of historical approaches tailored to each new health threat.

KEY POINTS FROM PART 1

- Public health measures and interventions made an important contribution to the decline in rates of mortality, including infant mortality, from the second half of the nineteenth century;
- The need for organised health provision came as part of increased urbanisation and communal living;
- The response to industrialisation and move to sanitation was implemented differently in different countries due to cultural, societal, historical, economic and political factors. It was initially based on the need for economic efficiency rather than concern for the conditions of the poor in society;
- The introduction of public health measures was not smooth. Change took time to achieve and was frequently met with resistance;
- The scope, focus and motives behind public health measures shifted according to political, social and economic need in each time period;
- Philanthropic individuals, associations, scientists and doctors played their part in the history of public health advances as well as governments, provincial and local authorities;
- The role of the State has been crucial in ensuring infrastructure and dedicated workforces are in place to bring about change;

DOI: 10.4324/9781003779902-6

- The interconnectedness of public health between countries and States in terms of mutual influence, interdependence and working together, and
- From the middle of the twentieth century there have been considerable efforts to coordinate response to major health issues internationally and globally.

The success of societies and their economies is ultimately dependent on a few factors, including, crucially, the health of their populations. The public health approach is well placed to help societies cope with future uncertainties in health because it aims to deal with the causes and not only the symptoms, treatment or consequences of disease.

SOURCES ACCESSED IN COMPILING PART 1

Berridge, V., *Public Health: A Very Short Introduction*, OUP, 2016.

Berridge, V., Gorsky, M. and Mold, A., *Public Health in History*, OUP, 2011.

Blake, J.B., 'The Origins of Public Health in the United States', *American Journal of Public Health Nations Health*, 38(11): 1539–50, November 1948.

Canadian Public Health Association, https://www.cpha.ca/history-public-health.

Chambaud, L. and Hernandez-Quevedo, C., *France*, Health Policy series no. 49, eds Rechel, B., Maresso, A., Sagan, A. et al., Copenhagen (Denmark) European Observatory on Health Systems and Policies 2018.

Druedahl, L.C., Minssen, T. and Nicholson Price, W., 'Collaboration in Times of Crisis: A Study on COVID-19 Vaccine R&D Partnerships', *Vaccine*, 39(42): 6291–95, 2 September 2021.

Edelstein, M., Lee, L.M., Herten-Crabb, A., Heymann, D.L. and Harper, D.R., 'Strengthening Global Public Health Surveillance through Data and Benefit Sharing', *Emerging Infectious Diseases*, 24(7): 1324–30, July 2018.

Edvinsson, S. and Nilsson, H., 'Urban Mortality in Sweden during the Nineteenth Century', in Brandstrom, A. and Tedebrand, L-G., eds. *Population Dynamics During Industrialisation* Demographic Data Base, Umea University, pp. 39–81, January 2000.

Gupta, Monica Das, *Public Health in India: An Overview*, January 2006, Working Bank Policy Research Working Paper No. 3787. papers.ssrn.com/S013/papers.cfm?abstract_id=873895.

Jones, D.S., 'The Persistence of American Indian Health Disparities', *American Journal of Public Health*, 96(12): 2122–34, December 2006.

Mackenbach, J.P., *A History of Population Health: Rise and Fall of Disease in Europe*, Clio Medical Online, Volume 101, Brill, 2020.

Marmot, M.G., Smith, G.D., Stansfeld, S. et al., 'Health Inequalities among British Civil Servants: The Whitehall II Study', *The Lancet*, 337(8754): 1387–93, 8 June 1991.

Mullen, J., 'History of Water Fluoridation', *British Dental Journal*, 199(7 Suppl): 1–4, 8 October 2005.

Mushtaq, M.U., 'Public Health in British India: A Brief Account of the History of Medical Services and Disease Prevention in Colonial India,' *Indian Journal of Community Medicine*, 34(1): 6–14, January 2009.

Porter, D. ed., *The History of Public Health and the Modern State*, Editions Rodopi B. V., Amsterdam-Atlanta, 1994.

Poscia, A., Silenzi, A. and Ricciardi, W., *Italy*, Health policy series no. 49, eds Rechel, B., Maresso, A., Sagan, A. et al., Copenhagen (Denmark) European Observatory on Health Systems and Policies 2018.

Rosen, G., *A History of Public Health*, The John Hopkins University Press, 1993.

Sachs, J.D. et al., *The Lancet Commission on Lessons for the Future from the COVID-19 Pandemic*, 400(10359): 1224–80, 8 October 2022.

Stewart, J., 'The "New Era in Medicine": John Ryle and the Promotion of Social Medicine', *Medical History*, 67(3): 247–65, July 2023.

Tichenor, M. et al., 'Interrogating the World Bank's Role in Global Health Knowledge Production, Governance and Finance', *Globalisation and Health*, 17(110), 2021.

Tulchinsky, T.H. and Varavikova, E.A., 'A History of Public Health', *The New Public Health* 3rd edn, pp. 1–42, Elsevier Academic Press, 2015.

For further information on the eradication of smallpox see:

Centers for Disease Control and Prevention (CDC), 'History of Smallpox', 23 October 2024. https://cdc.gov/smallpox/about/history.html?CDC_AAref_Val=https://cdc.gov/smallpox/history.history.html.

For further information on tobacco control legislation see:

Association of Directors of Public Health, 'The History of Tobacco Legislation', 9 June 2023. https://www.adph.org.uk/resources/the-history-of-tobacco-legislation.

PART 2

DEMYSTIFYING PUBLIC HEALTH

1 INTRODUCTION

There are many ways in which public health, the health of a population, can be changed for the better and, put simply, these are through efforts aimed at either improving health or at preventing disease. So let us start to demystify public health by introducing and explaining some terms that might otherwise be difficult before moving onto a description of the workforces and infrastructure that support delivery of public health initiatives and programmes.

The outline of Part 2 is as follows:

- health inequalities
- explaining public health terms
- the tools and knowledge available to be used for public health action
- the public health workforce and its underpinning infrastructure

2 HEALTH INEQUALITIES

First we should explore in more detail one conviction that underpins so much public health work, tackling health inequalities, and why it is so important to the public health community and to humanity.

I LIFE EXPECTANCY

One of the easiest ways to describe the impact of health inequalities is by looking at life expectancy.[1] In the UK, (looking at sex assigned at birth) women live longer than men on average, with a baby girl

DOI: 10.4324/9781003779902-7

expected to live an average of almost 83 years and baby boy 79 years, according to the most recent available data in 2025.[2] This gender difference is complex, but largely accounted for by higher infant (less than one year) mortality among boys and injuries due to accidents in young adult males.

If we then break down the life expectancy by where someone was born, we see, however, some big differences between areas of the country and even within cities and towns. For example, research back in the 1980s demonstrated graphically the loss in life expectancy going eastwards across London: in effect from affluent to poor suburbs. Little has changed. Using the latest data available (2021–23) a baby girl born in Barking and Dagenham is likely to live five years less than one born in Kensington and Chelsea. Her brother is likely to live five years less than a baby boy born in Richmond upon Thames.

We can look at the data in more detail to discover that *healthy* life expectancy differs, too: that is the number of years lived in good health. There is little difference in healthy life expectancy between males and females, but there remains the social gradient (whereby those living in more affluent areas generally live longer and in better health), so that both men and women in Lewisham typically have around 58 years of healthy life expectancy, compared with 70 years in Richmond upon Thames. Outside London, there persists a north-to-south gradient in life expectancy throughout the UK, with, for example, people in some parts of Glasgow still experiencing the short life expectancy at birth – less than 60 years – that more affluent parts of England experienced in Victorian times.

Inequalities exist internationally, too. Life expectancy is many years less in some low-income countries when compared with high-income countries.

II HEALTH INEQUALITIES AND ETHNICITY

Health inequalities are sometimes described by ethnicity and there is evidence in the UK that Black women are more likely than women of other ethnicities to die in pregnancy or childbirth. This disturbing finding is subject currently to formal investigation to address it. During the pandemic, marked differences in mortality were identified across different ethnic groups, some of which have been attributed to differences in lifestyle and family structure with multigenerational households, some to increased vulnerability due to metabolic disorders, but the apparent inequalities are not yet fully explained. Ethnic or racial inequalities are sometimes called disparities.[3]

III HEALTH INEQUALITIES AND THE DETERMINANTS OF HEALTH

Marmot described the 'causes of the causes' in his description of inequalities,[4] by which he meant the social determinants of health, which are the conditions in which people are born, grow, live, work, and age. Therefore, whilst personal behaviours, such as smoking, drinking alcohol or using street drugs, not getting much exercise and having a poor diet all contribute to ill health, these behaviours themselves are influenced heavily by the social determinants of health. The biggest single determinant is income, so that people who live in richer neighbourhoods are likely to be healthier on average, than those who live in poor areas.

Once you begin to think in this way, it becomes clear that if, for example, the streets around you are clean and safe, local shops sell fresh produce that you have enough money to buy because you have a decent job or pension, you are able to prepare meals in your kitchen at home, and because you understand that smoking is harmful to you and your family and have sufficient self-esteem to avoid smoking or other so-called 'bad personal habits', you are much better placed to live healthily than someone who achieved little at school, has a menial (or no) job with little satisfaction or status, lives on a dangerous housing estate, whose children cannot play outside, has living accommodation where you have no kitchen and in an area where you cannot access nutritious affordable food, and are suffering from stress that makes it hard to give up smoking or drinking. Recognising inequalities reflects wider societal values and is the flip side of simply blaming people as individuals for their bad habits, as if society has no responsibility for the opportunities or lack of opportunities in everyone's lives.

All these inequities lead to measurable differences in health status between different communities, dependent largely on income and other inequalities and the factors that emerge from them.

IV TACKLING HEALTH INEQUALITIES

Having discovered the causes – the underlying social determinants of health and ill health – you might think the solutions to health inequalities should be relatively easy to find and to make happen, but it is the case that, in the UK as in many other countries, inequalities are quite intransigent. Tackling them requires both the technical know-how (such as data manipulation, engaging communities, tailoring interventions) which we have, and the political will, which is only sometimes present. A recent previous Westminster government initiative aimed at 'levelling up' might have been expected to reduce social as well as health inequalities, but its implementation was patchy and the necessary investment to pull large numbers of people out of poverty was not forthcoming. Disappointingly, the present Labour government in the UK has so far taken few coherent steps to tackle social or health inequalities. We continue to see, therefore, gradients, some of them steep, in health experience between those who are relatively better off and those who are poorest.

V INEQUALITIES IN ACCESSING HEALTH CARE

People in countries that do not have a system of universal healthcare, free at the point of use, as we in the UK have enjoyed since 1948, tend to assume that we do not have health inequalities. After all, healthcare is free for everybody, correct? Actually no, at least some of the health inequalities we see in the UK are because healthcare is not equitably accessible to all of its residents. Although healthcare provision[5] is just one element in what determines the health of a population, lack of access to appropriate healthcare certainly contributes to health inequalities. For example, if you are a parent of several small children and you need to access care that is only available at the nearest hospital or clinic that might be a few miles away by public transport, you may make a legitimate, but sad decision that you cannot make the appointment, because the fare is high, the bus or train difficult, if not impossible, to access with a pram or double buggy and you have no-one with whom to leave your children or who can collect the eldest from school.

The language of health inequalities has to reverse terms like 'hard to reach' and ask difficult questions such as 'how to reach', how to help people to utilise health services. Continuing with the previous example, if the missed appointment is for a child's vaccination, then that child and their family and often their community, are at increased risk, compared with the vaccinated population, of falling seriously ill with a vaccine-preventable disease, which is what we see too often across towns and cities in the UK. Similarly, if the missed appointment was for cervical screening, that mother could be vulnerable to advanced cervical cancer, another disease that is largely preventable. These examples are indicative of a social gradient in many aspects of human health, with most diseases affecting the poorest members of society more severely than the rest of us. The social gradient in premature death reflects the outcomes of these differences in health experience.

Among more complex treatments that are often available only in large hospitals or centres of excellence, the same gradient can exist, because it is often the people who most need the service who are unable to access it. If, for example, you live in a mobile home in a semirural area, have no car and poor public transport, it is probable that you would be unable to keep an appointment at the major teaching hospital 50 miles away. Conversely, the affluent person who lives in the city and can easily drive or get a taxi to the same hospital, is likely to be able to access and therefore to benefit from that new or advanced treatment.

Such inequalities can sometimes be addressed relatively easily, for example, by the teaching hospital arranging with a local hospital to hold clinics there, but even this does not always capture all the patients who would benefit, because many of them would not yet have consulted their GP with their symptoms: we know that poorer people wait longer before seeking medical care, so they may be more unwell or have more advanced disease before they are seen by a doctor. This is one of the reasons we have high rates of cancer diagnosis in our Emergency Departments (or Accident and Emergency (A&E)) in the UK and efforts are being made to try to encourage people to seek medical advice sooner for a range of symptoms that could lead to earlier diagnosis and better outcomes.

Delivering healthcare differently has long been recognised as being necessary for everyone to have a fair chance to access it. So far, however, for a range of reasons – financial, logistical, capacity, lack of commitment, lack of political will – there remains rather often a 'one size fits all' mentality in healthcare, which is incompatible with truly universal coverage.

NOTES

1 Life expectancy at birth is the number of years a typical male or female baby can be expected to live depending on where they are born. In the UK in 2023, life expectancy at birth was just short of 79 years for males and 83 years for females.

2 https://www.ons.gov.uk/peoplepopulationandcommunity/birthsdeathsandmarriages/lifeexpectancies/bulletins/nationallifetablesunitedkingdom/2022to2024

3 Disparities is the term introduced to describe racial inequalities in the USA, now sometimes applied in the UK.

4 Institute of Health Equity, UCL, 11 November 2017. https://www.instituteofhealthequity.org/in-the-news/articles-by-the-institute-team-/inclusion-health-addressing-the-causes-of-the-causes---the-lancet-

5 See Dahlgren and Whitehead diagram on p.4.

4

EXPLAINING PUBLIC HEALTH TERMS

These terms have been selected as being both relevant for understanding public health and public health approaches. They are also widely used in briefings or press statements but possibly not fully understood.

1. OVERARCHING APPROACHES

I) PUBLIC HEALTH ISSUES

If a particular concern or problem impacts on the health and well-being of a population it can be described as a public health issue. This is a very wide definition and means that many issues which, at first or even second glance, do not seem anything to do with public health, are included. While it is obvious that a pandemic is a public health issue, since it clearly presents a threat to the health of the population affected, as are concerns about access to clean water and healthcare services, in recent decades other issues, such as natural disasters, air pollution, gun control, climate change and war, have all been identified as public health issues for exactly the same reason. To take just one of these examples, air pollution, there is now sufficient evidence that people living in areas where the air they breathe is continuously, or frequently, polluted, are more likely to suffer ill health or die prematurely.[1] Not only is this a public health issue, but also one that is associated with health inequalities, since those people most likely to be living in areas with poor indoor or outdoor air quality are also most likely to be the least affluent.

DOI: 10.4324/9781003779902-8

Tackling a public health issue may be approached in a variety of ways. In a society that prides itself on being liberal, responsibility is most commonly placed on the individual to resolve the issue, while in a more socially conscious society, responsibility may be taken by government or imposed on industry, to ensure improvements for the population rather than leave it to chance that individuals would take, or be able to take, the most appropriate actions.

II) HEALTH POLICY

Health policy is the way in which governments (at national, regional or local level) decide what action to take on matters of importance to the health of the population, such as the amount of funding for hospitals or GP practices or mental health provision (national), the capacity of substance misuse clinics or how to control outbreaks of infectious disease such as food poisoning (local).

The ways in which policy is made are numerous, but, if good practice is followed, then decision makers will apply the best available evidence to develop policy to address a specific issue facing their community. It follows that once policy is made, it will lead to a period of implementation to ensure that policy happens although, in practice, there may be a delay.

Usually, a new policy is announced only after research to confirm to policy makers that the policy will be welcomed by the people at whom it is aimed, who, in a political context, are often voters. In the event of a health emergency, such as a pandemic, however, policies intended to protect the public's health may have to be made and implemented rapidly and sometimes in the face of public opposition.

III) PREVENTION

The old adage that 'prevention is better than cure' remains true, but what does prevention really mean in the context of health and healthcare? Prevention takes a variety of forms, with the optimal form being *primary prevention*, in which something bad is stopped from happening before it begins. Straightforward examples of primary prevention include not being exposed to tobacco smoke as a means of not getting smoking-related lung cancer or other smoking-related disease, or retaining a healthy weight as the means of not getting obesity-related diseases.

The next type of prevention, *secondary prevention*, is similar, but further downstream towards disease, in that it is about identifying disease early enough to prevent the harm that would be done if the disease was allowed to progress unchecked. Probably the best-known example of secondary prevention is screening for some cancers and other serious conditions, where disease is detected at a very early stage in people who have no symptoms of the disease for which they are being screened. Screening-detected disease is usually diagnosed early, so that in most cases the most serious consequences of the disease are prevented.

Moving on to *tertiary prevention*, we see examples such as treating people with existing heart disease with statins for cholesterol or drugs to reduce blood pressure, in order to reduce the likelihood of more serious events such as a stroke or heart attack. Much of the talk on prevention that we see in healthcare in the 2020s is really about tertiary prevention, that is, interventions to keep people with serious long-term medical conditions out of hospital, preventing admissions by better community-based treatment and care. Whilst they have a value in shifting health care away from hospitals and closer to people's homes, these actions are not about the upstream changes that are necessary to prevent so many long-term conditions from starting in the first place.

IV) TIMING

It can take many years, if not decades, to bring about change in public health. Let us take the example of smoking in pubs (and other indoor public places). The evidence was clear and unambiguous that lives would be saved if people were not exposed to second hand smoke.[2] That idea was very unpopular with publicans, industry and with consumers, for pubs had, for centuries, of course, been places where customers smoked as they imbibed their beer or spirits. Only through a very carefully crafted, lengthy campaign engaging with a diverse range of different stakeholders did it become possible to gain the support of the public, the voters and then, of course, government ministers to what, at the time in 2007, was such a radical proposal leading to a change that now we all take for granted. Of note, in the first year after this legislation was passed, there were 1,200 fewer emergency hospital admissions for heart attacks.[3]

Had that legislation about smoking in enclosed indoor spaces been passed by government without the assent of the people, there would have been loud cries of '*Nanny State!*' In the event those cries were quite muted. The accusation of Nanny Statism is what happens when governments take unilateral action on issues that are for the public's benefit, before the voting public has indicated its readiness for change. Those who object most loudly are usually people who prefer a libertarian approach, with minimum interference from government. Commercial or other interests may be at play, too. A contemporary example subject to 'nanny state' accusations is the tax on alcohol (affecting minimum unit price or MUP). The evidence base indicates the poorest consumers are most likely to benefit most in terms of health but are also hardest hit by the price rise. Industry, the treasury and other interests have influence. At the time of writing, the Westminster government has yet to be persuaded to implement MUP in England, while it has become law in Scotland and Wales (with different minimum prices in each country).

If we consider the COVID-19 pandemic for a moment, the luxury of a lengthy period of public consultation about the rules needed to protect people and reduce the risk of death from the new virus was absent. Decisions had to be made rapidly, applying the best available evidence, and in the public interest. Mistakes were doubtless made, and a national public inquiry has recently published its second report, more of which later. But the ensuing rules that carried the nation – and indeed virtually all the world's nations – were imposed top-down by government in 'nanny state' style: not because governments wanted to adopt that style, but because that was essential to handle the emergency at the time. Regarding public health we sometimes refer to '*command and control*', a top-down autocratic system, which is more usually applied to military operations: but in some civil emergencies, such as a serious, rapidly spreading pandemic, the evidence shows that the most effective model for communicable disease control is the 'command and control' model.

V) BEHAVIOUR CHANGE

Part of the armoury of a public health worker is the knowledge of how to modify behaviour that has an adverse effect on health such as smoking, lack of exercise and poor diet. This can entail working with an individual or community. The approach will need to take in the wider context – income, employment, housing and education – and understand how these factors influence behaviour. Changing risky behaviour to adopting healthier activities involves complex interactions, for example, between an individual's own attitudes, interaction with others and the environment he or she lives in – at home, school, work, leisure or elsewhere.

If people are asked if they want to be healthy, they normally say 'yes'. In real life, however, people may continue to act in ways that are detrimental to their own health or that of their family. Health education or promotion interventions aim to help people live healthier lives. Typically, these interventions are aimed at individuals, but they may also be aimed at whole communities. Getting people to change their behaviour is not easy and is often made more difficult by the environments in which they live.

In the UK historically, there was a dependence on communicating health messages to the public via posters or advertisements in which the healthy options were described. Because these interventions often failed to take into account social and cultural differences in populations, these methods reached, appealed to, and were effective for, principally a certain group of people, typically those who were well educated and at least moderately affluent. Those people who were least well educated, and with the greatest risk of chronic ill health, who, therefore, had most to benefit from changing their behaviour, were largely excluded. This type of messaging failed them.

Campaigns to encourage people to eat more healthily fail miserably, around residential areas sometimes described as 'food deserts', where it is impossible to buy fresh fruit and vegetables.

The discovery that many health promotion interventions could, in practice, increase health inequalities prompted further research and policy solutions, to try to tackle the dilemma. Interventions such as 'Nudge' were tried by the Conservative-Liberal Democrat Alliance in the 2010s, having been effective in commercial marketing, whereby people were repeatedly prompted to take a particular course of action. This transfers to a social media approach to engage the public at scale.[4]

Population based interventions, particularly tailored to suit specific segments of society, are more likely to reap rewards because they can take into account the different, and often conflicting, factors that will affect the outcome. This means working with a community to understand what that whole community would need in order to embrace change, rather than imposing change or making suggestions in a vacuum. A combination of co-designed interventions may then be required and merely imparting information will rarely be sufficient.

In a neighbourhood where there is no fresh produce on sale, an approach working in partnership with communities would take on board the community's obvious need for fresh food to be available for sale locally, but could also include other changes to meet some of the needs they express, such as making safer the roads to the shops or providing cookery lessons. Other measures which might benefit the general health and wellbeing of the whole community, and not just individuals' behaviour, include ensuring safe outdoor play spaces.

Recent models of behaviour change are drawn from psychology and influenced by sociology and economics.[5] Goalsetting, action planning, regular prompting, self-monitoring, provision of incentives, disincentives, building a mindset for an active lifestyle may all be important for individuals, as well as motivational interviewing to help people explore their own decision making. The use and presentation of relevant data, consultation and involvement, the provision of rewards, supportive networks, setting community goals or use of social media may all help encourage positive behaviour in communities. Public health workers should be trained in the latest evidence and practice of what works best in which situations so that they can help to construct the most appropriate solutions. They do this in partnership with, and drawing on, the innate assets of the local community.

VI) LADDER OF INTERVENTION

Throughout history, in all societies, people acted in ways learnt from their parents and elders. What can or should be done, therefore, when it is discovered that some of those actions are bad for people's health? There are several possible strategies. One model to describe this array of possible interventions is known as the Intervention Ladder, developed by the Nuffield Council on Bioethics in 2007.[6]

As the baseline, there is do nothing other than share the information in a way that people will understand, and some may choose to modify their behaviour.

Moving up, you can make it easier for people to make healthier choices by all sorts of options, such as subsidy or other incentives. Going further, the State might get involved, and regulate or legislate for people to change their behaviour.

A criticism of the Ladder of Intervention is that its focus is on the behaviour of individuals rather than on the conduct of major industrial and other commercial players, where government intervention could be crucial in improving the health of the population.

VII) SOCIAL JUSTICE

Another concept that is central to public health is that of social justice, whereby there is an expectation that decisions made by society will be fair. For example, social justice may be demonstrated by policies that are fair and make no distinction between people on the basis of disability, ethnicity, sex, gender, age, sexual orientation or religion. The principles of social justice, since the nineteenth century, may be summed up as access to resources, equity, participation, diversity and human rights. In Victorian times, those people likely to benefit most from the State or charitable assistance were deemed to be either 'deserving' or 'undeserving', but such outdated value judgments have no place in modern society. Even so, today there still may be more public sympathy for some needy people than for others, emphasising the requirement for fairness by those in authority.

This goes well beyond health but given the centrality of health to the wellbeing of nations, social justice is a concept core to the achievement of optimal public health.

2. UNDERSTANDING HEALTH AND DISEASE

I) DETERMINANTS OF HEALTH

We touched on the determinants of health on p. 55 and in the introductory chapter in the Dahlgren and Whitehead diagram (p. 4). The determinants of health are those factors in our everyday lives that influence our health, both as individuals and as communities. Whilst it is obvious that healthcare provision and access to clean water are determinants of human health, it might not be so obvious that there are many other determinants, including income (and, conversely, poverty is a determinant of poor health), educational attainment, what we eat, our living environment (including housing and the external environment), how physically active (or inactive) we are, whether or not we drink alcohol or smoke or maintain a healthy weight, these are all determinants of health.

Recently, the concept of determinants of health has been expanded by the introduction of '*commercial determinants*', a term that is normally reserved to refer to those industries that are detrimental to health, including tobacco and alcohol, as probably the best known examples, but also fossil fuels, arms and those elements of the food industry that have led to huge consumption of ultra-processed foods, fast foods, and the consequent loss for many people of the constituents of a healthy diet. We now recognise commercial determinants of health as so critical to our health in the twenty-first century.

II) COMMUNICABLE DISEASES

Communicable diseases (CDs) are those medical conditions that can be spread from person to person, like measles, the common cold, COVID-19 and many more. Communicable diseases are caused mostly by tiny organisms that cannot be seen by the naked eye, including bacteria and viruses. Where an infection is carried in the breath, like the virus causing the common cold, for example, the patient can spread their infection by speaking or coughing when close to others, or where the infectious agent (bacterium or virus) sits in open skin lesions or spots, the infectious agent can be spread by touch.

Then there are other communicable diseases that cannot be transmitted from person to person, but via another means, often another animal. Probably the best-known example is malaria, which is spread by the bite of an infected anopheles mosquito, carrying the infected blood of one person to another. Sometimes the other means is an inanimate object, called a *fomite*, so that some diseases can be spread by the use of contaminated surgical instruments or by the dirty gloves or hands of a doctor or nurse. A brilliant example of our understanding of the spread of communicable diseases was provided by Ignaz Philipp Semmelweis, a Hungarian physician and scientist. He observed, as a junior doctor in Vienna in 1847, that many healthy women died unexpectedly with fever after childbirth, but that the number of women dying was much greater in the maternity unit staffed by doctors compared with the one staffed by midwives. It wasn't that midwives were inherently safer than doctors, it was that the doctors also attended post-mortem examinations and were exposed to infections that they subsequently brought with them to the maternity unit on their unwashed hands. Like many wonderful discoveries, it was before its time and was rubbished by the senior doctors of Semmelweis' time and only appreciated many years after his death, when the 'germ theory' of communicable diseases was accepted. Hand washing became the most important measure for infection control in hospitals and other healthcare settings, and whilst sterile gloves add further protection, simple, thorough hand washing with soap and water remains paramount.

There are also blood-borne and sexually transmitted infections where ordinary social interaction cannot cause spread of infection, but blood transfusion or intimate contact, respectively, can. HIV is an example of a virus that can be spread by both of these means, which, before that was recognised, caused the spread of infection to many thousands of people, most of whom died of AIDS or AIDS-related conditions in the 1980s and 1990s, before effective antiviral therapies were developed. Now, in the third decade of the twenty-first century, we have both antiviral therapies and effective measures for prevention of spread of the virus, as well as a much better-informed general public.

You might have noticed we have not used the term 'infectious disease' in this section. The reason for that is that you could have an infectious disease, a disease caused by an infectious agent, that is not a communicable disease. That would then just confuse everyone, because, of course, they behave like the non-communicable diseases below.

III) NON-COMMUNICABLE DISEASES

Non-communicable diseases (NCDs) are often described, not entirely accurately, as modern diseases or diseases of affluence, because they have become recognised as major causes of ill health and death in populations all over the world since most communicable diseases became treatable with the introduction of effective infection control measures and drugs such as antibiotics.[7]

NCDs largely comprise serious common diseases that we have all heard of – stroke, diabetes, cancers, respiratory and coronary heart diseases. Before the 1970s, most of these diseases were considered to afflict the more prosperous in UK society, with the image of the stressed, hard-working city type succumbing to a heart attack in middle age. The work of Sir Michael Marmot and colleagues changed that when, in 1987, he published his first of two reports on the Whitehall Study, a very large, long term study of English civil servants, in which it emerged that it was not the senior people who were most likely to succumb to these diseases in middle age, it was the least well paid and most junior civil servants, who often had least control over their working lives.[8]

The majority of common non-communicable diseases that cause many deaths annually in the UK affect those on low incomes and living in poor areas more than those people who are more affluent.[9] These medical conditions are usually described as long-term or chronic, though they may result in an acute or sudden life-threatening event such as a heart attack or stroke.

NOTES

1 Poor air quality is the largest environmental risk to public health in the UK, as long-term exposure to air pollution can cause chronic conditions such as cardiovascular and respiratory diseases, as well as lung cancer, leading to reduced life expectancy. https://www.gov.uk/government/publications/health-matters-air-pollution/health-matters-air-pollution.

2 Passive smokers suffer an increased risk of a range of smoking-related diseases. Exposure to other people's smoke increases the risk of lung cancer in non-smokers by 20–30% and coronary heart disease by 25–35%. https://ash.org.uk/resources/view/secondhand-smoke#:~:text=In%20the%20longer%2Dterm%2C%20passive,disease%20by%2025%2D35%25.

3 Sims, M., Maxwell, R., Bauld, L. and Gilmore, A., 'Short-term Impact of Smokefree Legislation in England: A Retrospective Analysis on Hospital Admissions for Myocardial Infarction', *British Medical Journal*, 340, 8 June 2010.

4 The Coalition Government under David Cameron set up the Behavioural Insights Team in 2010 which used 'nudge' theory.

5 https://assets.publishing.service.gov.uk/media/5a7f0d5940f0b6230268d23a/Behaviour_change_reference_report_tcm6-9697.pdf.
6 https://www.nuffieldbioethics.org/publication/public-health-ethical-issues/.
7 Some antibiotics are no longer effective in tackling drug-resistant bacteria in part due to the overuse of these drugs.
8 Marmot, M.G., Smith, G.D., Stansfield, S., Patel, C., North, F., Head, J., White, I., Brunner, E., Feeny, A., 'Health Inequalities among British Civil Servants: The Whitehall II Study', *The Lancet*, 337(8754), 1387–93, June 8 1991.
9 Between 2014 and 2016, as a cause of death, heart disease was the biggest contributor (1.49 years) to the difference in male life expectancy between the most and least affluent, followed by lung cancer (0.93 years) and chronic lower respiratory diseases (0.92 years). Between 2014 and 2016, as a cause of death among the most deprived females, chronic lower respiratory disease was the biggest contributor (1.04 years) to the difference in life expectancy, followed by lung cancer (0.86 years) and heart disease (0.82 years). https://www.gov.uk/government/publications/nhs-health-check-programme-review/annex-c-data-on-the-distribution-determinants-and-burden-of-non-communicable-diseases-in-england.

5

THE TOOLS AND KNOWLEDGE NEEDED FOR PUBLIC HEALTH ACTION

As we saw in the introductory chapter, public health is a combination of 'science' and 'art'. Here we look at what this means in terms of technical and general skills and knowledge used mainly by those in the public health workforce to influence, generate policy and run programmes. To deliver public health functions, public health workers will need a set of specific skills backed by in-depth knowledge. These are acquired through courses and field experience. The following are current in the UK, but many will be common to other countries as well. This section presents more examples of how and why a particular skills set and knowledge base are vital to the public health workforce as they carry out their activities to promote health, reduce inequalities and prevent disease.

1. SCIENCE

I) EPIDEMIOLOGY

Most people who study public health learn about the basic science called epidemiology. Epidemiology is about counting – people, events, cases of diseases. It is about understanding the occurrence, distribution, and possible actions needed for the control of diseases and other factors relating to health. Historically, epidemiology was all about infectious or communicable diseases, that is, about outbreaks or *epidemics*, but in the twenty-first century, it can be applied to any disease or medical condition.

DOI: 10.4324/9781003779902-9

Epidemiology is essentially the study (scientific, systematic, and *data-driven*) of the *distribution* (frequency, pattern) and *determinants* (causes, risk factors) of health-related states and events (not just diseases) in specified populations (for example, community, school, hospital, city, region, country, global).

It looks at how often diseases occur in different groups of people and why. Epidemiological information is used to plan and evaluate strategies to prevent illness and as a guide to the management of patients in whom disease has already developed.

Epidemiological information can be as important as clinical medical and pathological findings. Perhaps the best-known example is the link between cigarette smoking and lung cancer. This was discovered as a result of painstaking collection of data about patients being treated for lung cancer over many years, to establish patterns of the disease and possible causes, which led ultimately to confirmation of the causal link with smoking.[1]

Epidemiology can be used to explore an unlimited spectrum of conditions, so, for example, it came to the public's notice during the COVID-19 pandemic, when, in 2020, we watched the data about the pandemic on the Chief Medical Officer's graphs that were presented on television at the daily briefings. By following the distribution and numbers of cases, experts were able to *model* likely changes in the pandemic, although modelling – estimating things on the basis of mathematical calculations – is not always as accurate as we would like it to be. This was a factor that was particularly important during the pandemic, when there was no historical evidence about how that newly discovered virus might behave nor how best to treat people suffering from infection.

II) HEALTH INTELLIGENCE

Information is the lifeblood of any public health worker. As we have seen in Part 1, in the early days of modern public health, statistics on deaths, mapping of disease outbreaks, information on living conditions were all vital to understanding and making appropriate changes in infectious disease management.

Without relevant information today it would be impossible to provide accurate advice on health needs, risks to health, changes in populations which might have an impact on health, trends in and patterns of illness over time, and outcomes for different groups in the population or for the whole population. These data can be used to establish whether there are inequalities in acquiring specific illnesses or measures of ill-health, which will then allow policy makers to take appropriate decisions on service provision.

a) Information

By information we are referring to the collection, analysis and interpretation of data on health. This could take several forms, such as:

- establishing the number of people with a specific illness – or at risk of having a specific illness – in a specified geographical area, mapping their ethnicity, age and sex and ease of access or use of services to decide what services to provide and the best location for them;
- part of an *assessment of health needs* in relation to a particular health problem in a specified population;
- looking at risk factors or behaviours that may influence health adversely, such as smoking, enumerating the populations who smoke/do not smoke and any differences by age, sex, living and social conditions to inform further action to address the problem;
- in disease outbreaks such as food poisoning, establishing data on who is affected, who might be at risk of falling ill, locating and tackling appropriately the source of the food poisoning, so that further spread can be limited, appropriate treatment provided for those affected, while those still at risk but well are prevented from becoming ill;
- monitoring uptake and gathering data on at-risk groups who could be contacted or targeted for screening or immunisation.

b) Surveillance

Surveillance is a particularly important function of health intelligence. By the systematic regular collection, analysis, interpretation and communication of relevant data, it is possible to alert governments and the public to health and disease threats as well as monitor the impact of interventions.

c) Demographic information

Intelligence on life expectancy (the number of years that a person can expect to live, on average, in a given population), morbidity (the amount of disease within a population) and mortality (the number of deaths in a certain group of people in a certain period of time) are crucial in any collection of data describing a specific population. Collection, analysis and interpretation of this data can help determine risk factors of certain diseases and the effectiveness of certain health programmes. Crucially it can help identify the *incidence* (numbers of new cases) and *prevalence* (number of existing cases) of a particular disease or health issue in a defined population at a specific time.

Public health workers receive training in how and where to find relevant information, bringing together demographic and epidemiological data. This could include hospital and general practice data on the incidence and prevalence of a specific illness and service use, Census information on who is in local populations, their age and sex, information on deaths from death certificates. They then need to know how to analyse the data – taking care to ensure its accuracy and reliability – and interpret the results so that key messages on health, health trends and outcomes are clear and can be presented in understandable formats to a wide range of audiences who need to act on the information provided. It is worth mentioning here that use of personal data is protected in the UK by regulation and so data used for public health must generally comply with the requirements of General Data Protection Regulations (GDPR).[2]

In order to develop policies that will improve the health of a population, it is essential to understand the needs of that population and to be able to articulate them convincingly to policy makers. Reliable information is essential. The term *health needs assessment* (HNA) was coined to describe ways of understanding those needs and how best they can be met within available resources. Ways to do HNAs have evolved in the past few decades but, essentially, they aim to quantify a population's needs by looking carefully at the existing health of that population and then identifying the services required to address them. HNAs can be applied to a defined population's experience of a particular medical condition where outcomes could be improved, such as coronary heart disease, or more broadly to examine health care provision for a whole city.

III) HEALTH IMPACT ASSESSMENT

Health impact assessments (HIAs) are undertaken to look at the effects (the impacts both positive and negative) on health, usually of local people, of proposed new developments or changes to the environment, such as building a new factory, the redevelopment of a neglected inner-city area or a new transport system. The HIA can be used when a development is planned to maximise any health benefits from the change and minimise the harms.

The major Kings Cross development in London, started in 2008 but not completed until the 2020s, was subject to a major health impact assessment which looked at air quality during the construction period, the effect of the development on travel accessibility, and, in particular, the impact of the development on the local community socially and economically.

IV) UNDERSTANDING RISK

Understanding risk is important in public health, as in other aspects of life, as well as being a fascinating subject. It can easily be misrepresented, however. A classic example was the headline article in a Sunday newspaper in 1995.[3] It told women readers that their risk of dying because of taking the contraceptive pill was double compared with women who did not take the Pill.[4] What the paper omitted to tell their readers was the *absolute* risk: if someone who never took the Pill had a 1 in a million chance of dying, then a person who did take the Pill had a 2 in a million chance of dying: most people would probably take that risk! The *absolute* risk in this instance was very small indeed (1 in a million increasing to 2 in a million for pill takers). But the way the risk was described, as a *relative* risk, generated a huge amount of fear and meant that thousands of women stopped taking their Pill straight away, which, very unfortunately, led to a spike in unplanned pregnancies and greatly increased number of terminations.[5]

In November 2024, the NHS had a campaign to help people 'know your risk' of stroke due to high blood pressure. This used clear language to explain risk to the public and to encourage people to get their blood pressure checked, so that they could help themselves to reduce the risk where necessary.

The very straightforward take-away message is that when you read any story that talks about risk, check out whether it is describing relative risk – which very often can be misleading – or absolute risk, which nearly everyone can understand. That is not to say that any article about relative risk is intended to cause mayhem, but it does mean that authors, whether researchers, politicians or journalists, editors and publishers should be very careful and act responsibly.

V) EVIDENCE

Meeting health or healthcare needs requires application of *evidence*, so that the services put in place are most likely to be successful in solving the problem they are intended to address.

A central theme in striving to achieve good population health is to apply the best available evidence to the challenge to be addressed. Evidence is really a description of what we know about a topic. For example, when epidemiologists Richard Doll and Austin Bradford Hill presented the connection between smoking and lung cancer in 1954,[6] that was published as new evidence and subject to intense scrutiny within the academic and medical communities, as well as the general public. Longer term research showed conclusively that this was a causal relationship and not something that happened by chance. Despite this, it took a long time for the connection to be accepted.

VI) RESEARCH

High quality research is often essential in order to acquire the best evidence for making decisions.[7] Knowledge about, and experience in, carrying out well constructed research projects in public health are important underpinning skills to improving health. Without accurate research on, for example, the impact of air pollution on health, especially respiratory diseases, it would not be possible to establish what measure to put in place and where to locate smoke free zones.

Research on health can involve gathering information on populations and communities, as we have seen above, to inform local decision and policy making. This may be statistical information, or it could be small surveys and consultations with local communities. At the other end of the spectrum will be specific research studies, which may be short or long term, on particular health issues, diseases, health dilemmas for which answers are sought. These studies will have strict research protocols and methods to ensure the results are as robust and can be relied upon to inform subsequent action.

Public health workers are trained in a range of research methods – both quantitative and qualitative. Quantitative research looks at numerical data, answering questions such as 'how many' and 'how much' whereas qualitative research gathers information on people's experiences, perceptions and behaviour and answers questions such as 'how' and 'why'. Both approaches are essential in understanding how to improve health. Public health workers will also need to know which methodology to apply to answer a specific problem. Establishing whether a treatment is of benefit, for example, may call for a *randomised controlled trial* where one group of patients receives the treatment and a second receives a placebo but neither group knows which they have received. This is often described as the 'gold standard' in the world of evidence. It may be impossible to conduct such a trial in the real world, so we have then to turn to other types and sources of evidence.

Looking at the development of a particular disease in a certain group in the population may call for a long-term *cohort study* which follows the group over a period of years and tries to identify the factors that contribute to the onset of disease among those who are diagnosed or who die from the disease being studied.

Trying to understand barriers within a community to tackling a health issue might best be explored qualitatively, for example through a questionnaire seeking free text responses or through a series of structured or semi-structured interviews. This will include experiential evidence and opinion, which might come from experts or others, such as service users.

Research elicits evidence: over decades, a hierarchy of evidence has emerged, with some types of evidence carrying greater weight than others. However, the hierarchy is mainly applicable to quantitative methods, which may limit its application to public health research where qualitative and mixed methods are commonly used.[8]

VII) EVIDENCE REVIEW AND CRITICAL APPRAISAL

Findings from research are often published in scientific journals. Being able to find and review research findings and their authors' conclusions critically and judge the reliability of the information is an important skill for anyone interested in public health. It is essential to be able to locate, understand and interpret the research findings accurately. If advice is provided based on poor evidence the resulting policy or commissioning decision will usually be faulty. *Critical appraisal* means the ability to review the evidence on any topic and appreciate what it means in practical terms for the people or systems to whom it applies. Critical appraisal will explore the quality of evidence, how it is gathered, whether the ways in which the research was conducted (methodology) and results analysed were sound, whether the conclusions drawn were reasonable and the extent to which the published article is reliable and whether generalisations might be made from it.

Not everything that is published meets the highest standards we might expect. 'Do not believe everything you read' is important advice. Sometimes evidence is challenged, other times evidence can be used misleadingly. For example, Andrew Wakefield, a British gastroenterologist, and colleagues published an article in *The Lancet* in 1998 linking the MMR (measles, mumps and rubella) vaccine with autism. Researchers could not replicate his findings, and the article was eventually retracted in 2010 after the research had been exposed as fraudulent. Wakefield was erased from the UK medical register. This was too late to prevent loss of confidence among parents as well as an enduring anti-vaccination movement, which have led to repeated avoidable outbreaks of measles in the UK and elsewhere.

A particular use of evidence review is to look at what treatments work and on which patients. Is the treatment both effective in helping manage the disease or health problem and, secondarily does it present value of money? Some treatments may work but are deemed too expensive for the health benefit gained to be offered by the NHS. Based on such analyses, the National Institute of Health and Care Excellence (NICE) is responsible for advising the NHS on which treatments it should commission and provide.

VIII) EVALUATION

For any intervention tried or project undertaken it is essential to know whether it made a difference or not, and how. Was it safe? What worked? What did not work? What could be done better another time? Did it keep to the timetable? Was it within cost?

Safeguards to stop the intervention in the event of any suspicion of harm arising are essential. Evaluation needs to be set up from the outset, establishing the aims of the work, the key indicators that tell whether it is a success or not and measures put in place to track their progress. These could be quantitative (collecting numerical data) or qualitative (for example surveying recipients or professionals involved).

2. ART

The art of public health is what makes change happen. Numbers and science are essential but not sufficient. The art is about being able to present a picture in words and images that people will understand of how the world will look if public health action is implemented. Without the art of public health, people would still be smoking in pubs, driving without seatbelts and spreading preventable sexually transmitted infections. The *art* of public health is, therefore, about being able to translate the science into meaningful action, gaining traction for public health priorities to make a difference to people's health and wellbeing.

I) INVOLVING THE PUBLIC AND STAKEHOLDERS

A key element of the art of public health is being able to work successfully with members of the public and others to deliver change. A term often used in relation to public health, therefore, is *community and public engagement.* What is this and what might it achieve? In a functioning democracy, change normally happens through the assent of the people. If people are not helped to engage with their health, they will not necessarily respond favourably to changes for the good. About 25 years ago, a banker called Derek Wanless was asked by the government to review the health of the population in England and to advise how to do better: he introduced an important concept, '*the fully engaged scenario*', whereby ordinary people would be sufficiently interested in their own health to understand the factors that impact it. Because they had bought into the idea that it is important, they could see how actions by both government and themselves could result in improvements.[9] The concept of community engagement, whereby whole communities are partners in the co-design and delivery of interventions to improve their health is of critical importance. Community engagement recognises the assets brought to the task by the community itself. Using what may be described as an *assets-based* approach, it builds on the community's assets and does not view communities in need of help simplistically as part of – or even worse, as the cause of – the problem.

As well as community and public engagement, we also need to include *stakeholder engagement*. Obviously, communities are stakeholders, but this latter term is used more widely, embracing interests as diverse as industry, commerce, agriculture, education, and politicians, that is, all those who may need to be involved in decisions that influence the health of a population. Sometimes, public health workers are criticised for engaging with industries whose activities are harmful to health, but such engagement with difficult stakeholders offers, if carefully conducted, important, evidence-based challenges to those individuals or industries.

II) PARTNERSHIP WORKING

Because of the complexity of many programmes and initiatives, they often need input from a variety of players and organisations bringing complementary expertise and reach. Knowing how to work effectively in partnership with other individuals, groups or organisations is crucial.

Important in successful partnership working is identifying all the key stakeholders for any particular piece of work and making sure they are on board with the project. Partners can be engaged as part of a steering or advisory group for a project or to ensure delivery. In local projects it is important that they help shape programme delivery through their intimate knowledge of the community. Engagement and consultation at this point are crucial and require good listening and communication skills and an ability to adapt to the circumstances presented. A project to improve dental health among children by encouraging effective tooth-brushing in schoolchildren in a specific locality, for example, might include the local council, dentists, community leaders, school staff and parents as partners with the dental public health team.

III) GENERIC/TRANSFERABLE KNOWLEDGE AND SKILLS

a) Project and financial management

Public health workers are frequently called upon to set up and run or oversee specific projects from development through to completion and review. They will, therefore, need skills in project and financial management. These may include knowledge and experience of how to write a successful business plan, writing a project plan with goals, milestones, timescales, set up a steering group which includes all relevant partners in the project, organising a delivery team, having regular review points, allocating funding and monitoring its spend. Sometimes, projects can be enormously complex and involve several partners and delivery arms. All projects need *evaluation* to determine what, if anything, has changed. This will mean setting up relevant data collection methods from the outset to monitor change and being clear on the key measures that will indicate the extent to which project aims have been achieved.

b) Communication

Good communication – written and spoken on a variety of media – is vital for public health work. Every piece of communication should be for a purpose, so, for example, a press release to alert the public to a potential risk to health such as an increase in the incidence of an infectious disease might differ in format and content from the publicity put out on posters, leaflets or what is communicated through social media.

Much health communication is based on complex information. Therefore, it is important to know how to present information in a way that is understandable and relevant to a range of audiences, some expert but many not. Presenting the results of a research project to a professional audience at a conference will be very different to sharing local data with a meeting of councillors in local government. Consulting with local communities and working with their leaders will also require skills in engagement and listening.

Public health workers will, therefore, need to be practised in presenting information and consulting across a range of different audiences, formats and communities, and know how to convey relevant health messages successfully in each.

c) Leadership

Leadership in public health can also take various forms and does not always mean standing at the front and telling people what is expected and what to do. Effective public health intervention requires knowledge of how to influence at all levels. This might mean working within local communities or, for example, convincing a local council to change its policy on fast food outlet licencing near schools, or it might mean influencing government to bring in a new policy on alcohol pricing. Those working in public health may frequently have to challenge the status quo and use information and evidence to back up their position and gain support from others.

Leadership in public health can also mean knowing when to take the lead oneself and when to allow others to take the lead, being prepared to be a team member, not necessarily always the leader. During the Coronavirus pandemic in the UK, the country got used to seeing the Chief Medical Officer directly advising the public how best to reduce their risk of infection. We also saw the Prime Minister and other Ministers taking the lead armed with information and evidence provided for them. We know that a trusted voice is likely to be most effective. When working with other agencies or organisations, the public health representative may lead on some aspects while others take the lead on other aspects to achieve the desired outcome. All this needs flexibility and creativity in approach.

The public health team itself needs sound leadership. Good individual and team management skills are also, therefore, required to motivate, delegate and supervise others. The ability to build good working relationships is crucial.

When people working in public health refer to their work, they often talk about the passion that drives them to make the world a healthier place. It is this passion which is frequently communicated in their manner of leadership and which will encourage others. Passion and a degree of resilience to withstand challenge are key characteristics of good leaders.

d) Ethical and legal practice

Public health workers are required to abide by a code of conduct which includes adhering to ethical behaviour. The UK Faculty of Public Health's *Good Public Health Practice* [last updated 2024] outlines the duties, responsibilities, competence and behaviour expected of a professional working in public health.[10]

A core principle of medical and public health ethics is autonomy, which is often described as the right to self-determination. An appreciation of public health ethics and their relationship with medical and healthcare ethics is important to everyone involved in public health systems. Ethical practice for clinicians includes 'doing no harm' and acting 'in the best interests' of patients. Public health ethics crucially apply to whole communities or populations, rather than having their focus on the individual. Public health ethics embrace fairness and optimal use of scarce resources for the benefit of the whole population, applying to the community as a whole the principles of doing no harm and acting in best interests.[11]

Public health normally operates within a legal framework, most commonly that of the nation where the public health organisation is based. These frameworks vary markedly between countries, with some including quite draconian disease control measures, for example, while others have not introduced such restrictions. During the Coronavirus pandemic, we saw great variation in the application of laws affecting institutions and individuals. For international organisations to function, the laws of several jurisdictions may need to be heeded. International Health Regulations play an important function globally.[12]

e) Technological tools

The benefits of technology have transformed access to the information that is central to public health action, particularly in recent years. Aids range from support to individuals to large data sets and surveillance systems. Digital information, for example, can allow for more refined stratification of population health-related data by time, place and personal characteristics which, in turn, can lead to greater precision in the public health response.

Particularly since the pandemic, there has been a large increase in mobile phone devices and applications, location tracking technologies, temperature scanning and wearable devices such as for contact tracing. Downloadable apps from the NHS, to help individuals looking to monitor or change their lifestyles, cover quitting smoking, drink free days, promoting exercise, scanning barcodes for sugar and salt content of food purchased.[13]

The Department of Health and Social Care in England operates Fingertips, a large public health data collection, organised in themed profiles, with indicators showing local area data alongside relevant comparative health trends.[14] The health inequalities dashboard for England includes, for example, the following indicators: the prevalence of obesity, smoking rates and the numbers of 16–17 year olds not in education.[15]

The UK Health Security Agency (UKHSA) has a digital dashboard with data on COVID-19, influenza and other respiratory illnesses.[16] It also has a real time syndromic[17] surveillance team (ReSST) which collects and analyses anonymous health data from several sources, looking for trends including higher than usual occurrence of infectious illness, and publishes bulletins to keep public health professionals up to date.[18]

3. EVIDENCE INTO ACTION

Competence – knowledge and skills – is of little use if it cannot be applied to practical action. Before any public health programme can be implemented, there has to be preparation and understanding of the current situation and defining the current problem to be addressed, what the aims are and what needs to change to achieve these aims. So, conducting a health needs assessment is one activity that utilises a broad range of public health competencies. To complete such assessments, those working in the public health field will need to review relevant service data and demographical information to establish the current situation, consult widely with local people, organisations and workforces to establish views on what the issues are, establish the evidence of what works in that particular situation, and engage with local stakeholders to work out what, practically, can be delivered and when.

NOTES

1 Doll, R. and Bradford Hill, A., 'The Mortality of Doctors in Relation to their Smoking Habits: A Preliminary Report', *BMJ*, 1, 1451, 26 June 1954.
2 GDPR: General data protection regulation. For further information see: https://www.gov.uk/data-protection
3 *The Sunday Times Magazine*, 19 November 1995.

4 In October 1995, the UK Committee on Safety of Medicines had issued a warning about an increased risk of venous thromboembolism in women taking certain oral contraceptives. The warning was based on unpublished studies that suggested a doubling of the risk. The warning was released before the scientific papers were published.

5 Furedi, A., 'Social Consequences. The Public Health Implications of the 1995 'Pill Scare', *Human Reproduction Update*, 5(6), 621–26., 1 November 1999

6 Doll and Bradford Hill, 'The Mortality of Doctors in Relation to their Smoking Habits'.

7 There are cautions in using AI for research evidence – incomplete or biased data, inaccurate information etc.

8 https://www.healthknowledge.org.uk/public-health-textbook/research-methods/1a-epidemiology/hierarchy-research-evidence

9 https://si.easp.es/derechosciudadania/wp-content/uploads/2009/10/4.Informe-Wanless.pdf. Wanless, D., *Securing our Future Health – Taking a Long-term View: The Wanless Report*, HM Treasury, 17 April 2002.

10 https://www.fph.org.uk/news/uk-faculty-of-public-health-launches-latest-edition-of-good-public-health-practice/ 7 October 2024. This updates its 2016 Good Public Health Framework.

11 https://www.fph.org.uk/public-health-ethics-and-law/

12 https://www.who.int/health-topics/international-health-regulations#tab=tab_1

13 https://www.nhs.uk/better-health/

14 https://fingertips.phe.org.uk/profile/health-profiles

15 https://analytics.phe.gov.uk/apps/health-inequalities-dashboard/

16 https://ukhsa-dashboard.data.gov.uk/about

17 A group of signs and symptoms that occur together and characterize a particular abnormality or condition.

18 https://www.gov.uk/government/collections/syndromic-surveillance-systems-and-analyses

6

THE PUBLIC HEALTH WORKFORCE AND THE INFRASTRUCTURE TO SUPPORT IT

1. INTRODUCTION

To deliver change in population health we need structures and organisation for strategy, policies and specific programmes to be developed and a workforce to inform those strategies and policies as well as delivering consequent programmes. In turn, this workforce will need knowledge and skills, brought about through specific training and backed by technology to carry out their work. We will, therefore, focus here on the underpinning organisations, workforce, training and tools to support public health action to improve and sustain the health of populations and communities.

As we have seen in Part 1, the workforce delivering public health action has changed and broadened over the years, along with our understanding of population health issues. As might be expected, given the complexity of current health priorities, the workforces tackling them are numerous and varied and will include those with backgrounds in medicine, nursing, environmental health, data handling, epidemiology, programme management, communications, teaching, health promotion, pharmacy, psychology, social science and research.

Although countries will have workforces delivering public health functions and universities all over the world offering degree courses in public health, there is no universal description or single definition of 'public health' as a term for the workforce. The personnel involved and their nomenclature will differ from country to country depending on historically how responsibility for the public's health has developed. Even the medical specialty of public health is identified

DOI: 10.4324/9781003779902-10

by different titles – hygiene and preventive medicine in the Czech Republic, for example, and social medicine in Sweden.

In some countries, the public health workforce is primarily medically led as in France, and also in Italy where it forms part of the healthcare service.[1] In the United States, from early days as we have seen, it has been multidisciplinary.

There may be no separate or dedicated public health service. Services are frequently run from municipalities with a range of staff, or form part of health care where health service staff carry out public health functions.

This is primarily a dispersed workforce. Where people are based will differ in different countries, depending on how health, social care and other related services are organised and funded, and where responsibility for delivering public health functions currently lies. This could be at national level, regional level or the very local level in society, in public, privately funded, or charitable organisations.

Training will also vary from country to country, whether at Master's, bachelor's degree or diploma level, multidisciplinary or single specialty. Schemes may be nationally provided or nationally accredited or neither. For many countries, there may be no specific specialist training programmes.

Because of this complexity, this chapter will concentrate on the public health workforce in the UK, as the example. We will begin with an outline of the common functions of the public health workforce before looking at structures.

2. WHAT THE PUBLIC HEALTH WORKFORCE DOES

While structures, and how the workforce might be described and operate, differ across the world, the aims are universal, to improve health and reduce inequalities.

Functions have changed and widened since the middle of the nineteenth century when the focus was primarily on providing clean water and sewerage and improving urban environmental air quality.

The UK Faculty of Public Health[2] in May 2024 outlined the following priorities for the workforce to promote the public's health:

1. Promote policies and programmes that improve the health and wellbeing of people and communities and tackle health inequalities.

2. Tackle poverty to ensure everyone has the chance to live a long and healthy life.
3. Protect the nation from infectious diseases and prepare for health threats and emergencies.
4. Increase investment in public health and prevention as assets for society and make health a priority for cross-government action.[3]

To fulfil these objectives, most people working in public health will focus on one or more of the following three broad areas of practice:

a) Improving health – by this we mean working to boost people's health and wellbeing and help prevent ill-health and disease. Examples could be smoking legislation at the national level or advising individuals on how to make changes to their lifestyle such as advocating healthy eating, stopping smoking or taking regular exercise; working with communities on specific campaigns such as promoting safer sex; running screening programmes such as for breast and cervical cancer.
b) Protecting health – by this we mean working to ensure the safety of the population. Examples could be protecting people from infectious diseases such as during an outbreak of meningitis or food poisoning by tracing the origins of the infection, organising treatment and ensuring the public is aware of the risks and how to avoid them; protecting people from what we call environmental hazards such as chemical or radiation leaks, excessive noise; ensuring restaurants and food manufacturers adhere to regulated hygiene standards.
c) Maintaining and raising standards of health and social care – by this we mean working to improve outcomes for patients or clients and ensure the services provided are safe, efficient and effective. Examples could be informing the commissioning of those responsible for letting contracts for health care; setting priorities for services based on the best evidence of what treatments work matched to the health needs of specific populations such as the very elderly, children or specific ethnic groups, vulnerable or disadvantaged communities; advising on the quality and safety of services and evaluating whether the services are delivering what they should be doing.

Across these three areas of practice, those working in public health may also be involved in developing national, regional or local policy, collecting, analysing and interpreting information, evaluating specific programmes or undertaking research to further knowledge on particular issues and establish what might work to improve health.

The Royal College of Physicians (RCP), in collaboration with a number of health and public health organisations, issued in 2025 a set of principles for an effective integrated public health system. This emphasises the need for public health to be embedded in and joined up across national, regional and local organisations, with decisions based on shared public health goals. Public health skills and leadership should be valued and those working in public health should act in collaboration.[4]

3. THE UK PUBLIC HEALTH WORKFORCE AND ITS STRUCTURE

In England, the Department of Health and Social Care, accountable to the Secretary of State for Health, is responsible for public health. Those working in public health in England will be based in a range of different organisations depending on the function they are delivering and at which level, whether national, regional or local. Many public health professionals will work in local government councils, delivering local health improvement and some health protection services as well as providing input to health care commissioning. A few will be employed within NHS hospital and community services providers to promote evidence-based decision making and inform the delivery of front-line services. Health is a devolved function in Wales, Northern Ireland and Scotland, which all have their own national public health agencies which employ most public health staff.

There are a number of agencies at the national level employing staff working on public health such as the government UK Health Security Agency (UKHSA), which also has regional departments, and which is focused on health protection. Another is the Office of Health Improvement and Disparities (OHID) which is part of the Department of Health and Social Care (DHSC). In addition, public health personnel can be found in charitable organisations aiming to influence health policy, public health academics in university departments, consultancies, voluntary bodies and NGOs.[5]

The UK public health workforce can be described by dividing it into three groups: specialists, practitioners and what we call the 'wider workforce'. Let us explain this further.

I) SPECIALISTS

Public health specialists tend to work at senior management or strategic levels, leading programmes and teams. They have usually undergone specific training over a number of years to achieve qualification as a consultant and be registered with one of the UK's three specialist public health regulatory bodies.[6] Crucially, most specialists are competent, on completion of their training, to work across all the public health functions outlined above. The UK is unusual in that applicants for these training schemes – and therefore for the consultant workforce – will come from both medical and other backgrounds. In the UK, specialist training is consistent, regardless of trainees' professional backgrounds.

Specialists form the smallest numerical group in the workforce. There are specific four-to-five-year training programmes in the UK for those aiming to become specialists. Following registration, specialists are obliged to continue to learn and develop to ensure skills and knowledge are up-to-date and they remain fit to practise, with regulators imposing five-yearly revalidation for individuals to demonstrate this, aimed at providing assurance to the general public.

II) PRACTITIONERS

Public health practitioners work at the operational level, that is delivering programmes on the ground. Many have professional qualifications in their specific area of practice and are subject to regulated practice, such as environmental health officers who work in the area of health protection, public health pharmacists, public health nurses, health visitors and midwives.[7] In addition, there will be public health managers and those with expertise in working with data and information. Many of these individuals will have relevant undergraduate or Master's degrees or have undergone a public health apprenticeship. Those practitioners who are in regulated professions are obliged to undertake ongoing development.

This is the second largest group in the workforce.

III) WIDER WORKFORCE

This is the largest and most diffuse group and includes many people who would not necessarily describe themselves as working within the sphere of public health but who, through their roles, nevertheless contribute to improving health and wellbeing in the population and reducing inequalities. Within this broad workforce could be head teachers working to educate and support disadvantaged children in their catchment areas, social workers striving to improve the circumstances of poor families and isolated elderly people or those in the voluntary sector dealing, for example, with poor housing or homelessness. You can reflect on your own life in ways you might be already contributing or could help improve general health and wellbeing or reduce inequalities in the community around you.

The UK is unusual in having a public health competency framework which is applicable to all those working in the field, at whatever level, and describes the functions and activities of the workforce.[8]

For those interested in a career in public health in the UK, relevant websites are listed in the Part 2 Summary (p. 92). Given the challenges to health, the capacity to tackle them needs to grow. This means not only those formally trained in public health but those in the 'wider workforce' who need to be aware of their potential roles in improving health and equipped to contribute as never before.

4. EXAMPLES OF THE WIDER INFRASTRUCTURE IN THE UK

A key feature of the wider public health infrastructure are the Voluntary and Community Sector (VCS) Organisations. In the UK, charities frequently focus on one sector of the population (such as older people) or on a specific disability (eg learning disabilities) or medical condition (eg motor neurone disease). They are increasingly being used to provide essential support to the work of statutory agencies such as the health service and local government and are valued for their direct contact with the community. The voluntary sector makes extensive use of the wider public health workforce to deliver its services to support health improvement in particular and help tackle health inequalities. The voluntary sector also often has a role in advocacy for the group it represents, as well as lobbying and campaigning for additional funding and service change. Some larger charities may have research sections. Some organisations are lobbying groups for particular disease areas or health issues, such as Action on Smoking and Health (ASH).

National independent policy '*think tanks*' such as The King's Fund and the Health Foundation act to influence policy for health and service improvement for all. By undertaking research, producing evidence-based reports and papers they may challenge or endorse existing policy and promote policy change.

NOTES

1 https://www.ncbi.nlm.nih.gov/books/NBK507328/; https://www.ncbi.nlm.nih.gov/books/NBK535727/
2 The professional organisation for public health specialists, a faculty of the UK's Royal Colleges of Physicians.
3 https://www.fph.org.uk/policy-advocacy/what-we-think/a-vision-for-the-publics-health/
4 https://www.rcp.ac.uk/policy-and-campaigns/policy-documents/rcp-principles-for-an-effective-integrated-public-health-system
5 Public health structures are slightly different in Northern Ireland, Wales and Scotland. See Sim, F. and Wright, J. (eds), *Working in Public Health*, 2nd edition, Routledge, 2024, pp. 15–18.
6 Regulatory bodies for public health specialists: the General Medical Councils (for doctors), the UK Public Health Register (mainly for those who are not medically qualified), the UK General Dental Council (for those qualified in dental public health).
7 Regulatory bodies for public health practitioners include: the Chartered Institute of Environmental Health (CIEH), the Nursing and Midwifery Council (NMC) and the General Pharmaceutical Council (GPhC).
8 https://www.gov.uk/government/publications/public-health-skills-and-knowledge-framework-phskf/public-health-skills-and-knowledge-framework-august-2019-update

SUMMARY

Part 2 has sought to clarify and explain public health terms, emphasising their relevance in tackling population health issues. Equally important are the skills needed by those working in public health and the infrastructure to support them. It is a complex system with a diverse and diffuse workforce, unified in the UK by a common framework of competence and knowledge and a common drive to improve health and reduce health inequalities.

Most of the examples in this section have come from the United Kingdom. Around the world, the composition of public health workforces will vary as will the infrastructures to support them.

Wherever in the world public health workforces are operating, however, they will need not only to be competent but also flexible and adaptable to constantly changing circumstances and issues.

How these workforces are tackling some of the major health issues of our time will be explored in the next part.

USEFUL READING ON PUBLIC HEALTH TERMINOLOGY

Carr, S., Unwin, N. and Pless-Mulloli, T., *An Introduction to Public Health and Epidemiology*, OUP, 1997.

Dahlgren, G. and Whitehead, M., 'The Dahlgren–Whitehead Model of Health Determinants: Thirty Years on and Still Chasing Rainbows', *Public Health*, 199: 20–24, 2021. Accessed 12 December 2025 at: https://www.sciencedirect.com/science/article/abs/pii/S003335062100336X.

Schneider, M.J., *Introduction to Public Health*, Jones and Bartlett Publishers, 2000.

Wilson, F. and Mabhala, M. (eds), *Key Concepts in Public Health*, Sage, 2009.

DOI: 10.4324/9781003779902-11

USEFUL RESOURCES FOR THOSE INTERESTED IN A PUBLIC HEALTH CAREER IN THE UK

Chartered Institute of Environmental Health www.cieh.org
Faculty of Public Health www.fph.org.uk
General Dental Council www.gdc-uk.org
General Medical Council www.gmc-uk.org
NHS Health careers website www.healthcareer.nhs.uk/explore-roles/public-health-careers
Nursing and Midwifery Council www.nmc.org.uk
Public Health Skills and Knowledge Framework www.gov.uk/government/publications/public-health-skills-and-knowledge-framework-phskf/public-health-skills-and-knowledge-framework-august-2019-update
Royal Society for Public Health www.rsph.org.uk
Sim, F. and Wright, J. (eds), *Working in Public Health – Choosing the Right Career*, 2nd edition, Routledge, 2024.
UK Public Health Register www.ukphr.org

PART 3

CRITICAL CHALLENGES TO HEALTH

INTRODUCTION

This part of the book looks at global health challenges in the context of where the public health movement is now, moving into the second quarter of the twenty-first century. Previous sections have shown the history of public health to the present day, the knowledge and skills that tackle modern day challenges and, lastly, the structures within which public health workforces operate. This part serves to bring these previous parts together to illustrate how the public health issues of today are being tackled and what public health knowledge and skills might contribute in the future.

Out of the myriad of public health challenges that face the world today,[1] we have selected a few that present substantial challenges to the health of populations in a variety of contexts and for different reasons. The aim is to make the reality of public health recognisable, tangible and accessible.

Each chapter explains why these challenges are important to our lives and what some of the solutions might be. They illustrate the diversity of the issues and the contribution those working in public health can make.

For each challenge, however unique, the public health approach will be familiar, but is used flexibly, relying on a combination of knowledge, skills and perseverance we have described earlier. How these are deployed will be explored in each chapter.

For each challenge, there are similarities. The impact is felt most by the most vulnerable in society, widening health inequalities in most cases. For major issues there is often a need for collaborative

DOI: 10.4324/9781003779902-12

effort across countries, although the extent of international or global response varies. For tobacco control, for example, there is a commonly accepted international framework, and for control of pandemics, the International Health Regulations.[2]

The Chapter outline is as follows:

- the COVID-19 pandemic
- bodyweight
- tobacco control – halting the pandemic
- the future – challenges and opportunities

NOTES

1 War, terrorism, natural disasters, ageing populations, famine, infectious disease, lack of clean water to name a few.

2 The International Health Regulations (2005) provide the international legal framework for the prevention and response to the international spread of diseases. 1 January 2016. WHO https://www.who.int/publications/i/item/9789241580496

7

THE COVID-19 PANDEMIC

1. INTRODUCTION

One major recent challenge for the world has been living through the emergence and enormous impact of a new infectious disease. It will come as no surprise to readers to hear that the Coronavirus pandemic was also a huge challenge to public health.

In the UK, initially the pandemic brought an uncharacteristic consensus politically, with politicians across the spectrum showing a unity that was apparently reminiscent of wartime. For a while, the interests of the nation and of its people seemed to many to overrule partisan or personal interests, but that was short-lived and, in any case, there were exceptions, with some politicians exhibiting strong denial of conflicts of interest.

In the face of a pandemic caused by a newly discovered organism such as COVID-19, the starting point was an absence of evidence about what policies or interventions might work. There was a short-lived assumption by some that this pandemic would 'behave' like influenza, which turned out to be wrong. Other experts drew on experience with other recent pandemics caused by new organisms, notably SARS or MERS, but it became apparent, through early surveillance, that this pandemic would be different. From a public health perspective, this brought two contradicting emotions: the first, rising to the challenge of tackling such a momentous event, the second, profound fear that the tools to tackle this pandemic effectively would have to be developed more rapidly than ever before.

In such a situation where a contagious viral disease was causing serious illness, urgent hospital admissions and many deaths globally,

DOI: 10.4324/9781003779902-13

public health actions that could contribute to a lasting solution were needed at all levels – local, national, international. Public health solutions would usually be based on the best available evidence for a particular intervention, which might be a 'tried and tested' formula. Since this pandemic was caused by a new virus that behaved differently from most previously known pandemic organisms, there was little relevant experience on which to base solutions. Unlike other pandemics, there was no greater experience globally either, so that international organisations such as the WHO were not well equipped to lead the global response. The lack of robust evidence led, as we shall see, to diverse policies and interventions and many of these are still subject to evaluation.

2. THE BEGINNINGS OF THE PANDEMIC

The COVID-19 pandemic began, like any new infectious disease, as a local problem. In late 2019, reports were emerging from the city of Wuhan in China, about unusual cases of pneumonia, which were causing some otherwise healthy adults rapidly to become seriously ill or even to die. The virus causing this had not yet been identified when reports of something very similar began to come from South Korea, Iran and Western Europe. A common feature of some of that early inter-Continental spread was air travel, including skiing holidays. In the space of a few weeks, what had begun as a worrying local outbreak of severe respiratory illness had become an international incident. On 31 January 2020, the World Health Organization declared the outbreak a 'Public Health Emergency of International Concern' and then, on 11 March 2020, a (full-blown) 'pandemic'. By that date, cases had been reported in 114 countries, although 90% of cases were in just four countries, and more than 4,000 people had already died.

From the first recognition of an international outbreak, there was a need for local, national and international action to tackle the pandemic, with coordination and cooperation being essential at every level. The reality was rather different. Small local outbreaks of infectious diseases are normally handled by applying well-established, effective public health principles of communicable disease control[1] and are rarely newsworthy. Cultural differences, the opaque (to the outside world) nature of dealing with the original Chinese outbreak, the fact that this was a new communicable disease, as well as its severity and rapid spread in our modern connected world meant that the infection had become widespread by the time the rest of the world became fully aware.

We shall look in this chapter mainly at the UK experience. Like other countries, the UK had experience in managing outbreaks, epidemics and even pandemics,[2] but the plans that had been developed anticipated infections with viruses with which we were familiar and not the new or 'novel' Coronavirus: this was the world's first pandemic caused by a coronavirus. Policy and action to control the pandemic had to be reviewed, therefore, and adapted in real time as the behaviour of the virus became better understood.

3. ATTEMPTS TO CONTROL THE PANDEMIC

I) COMMUNICATION (AND SOME MISINFORMATION)

a) Official lines of communication

Clear communication and delegation are vital aspects of managing epidemics, which often require a 'command and control' military-type approach. As disclosed in the subsequent national review, local healthcare and public health leaders were not always kept aware of the parts they were expected to play, nor provided with resources to ensure safety of their local residents or of frontline health and social care workers and others at increased risk of exposure, such as those working in public transport or in retail. There were frequent complaints from the early days of the pandemic that major policy decisions were communicated to the local public health 'frontline' via the Prime Minister's daily televised update and not via normal professional or line management channels.

Despite the difficulties, communicating effectively with the public was of central importance during the pandemic. Whether at local level, in the (Local Authority) Council chamber, or on national television or in the press or on social media, it was important for the rational, sensible and objective public health voice to be heard. Nationally, England's Chief Medical Officer and Chief Scientific Officer were frequently heard in this role. At the more local level, Directors of Public Health (DsPH) became trusted voices. This was pointed out by the King's Fund which described DsPH as providing skilled leadership of the local response to COVID-19. This also helped to build trust among other stakeholders in health and care and local government.[3]

Communication about people's health is often targeted by libertarians as indicative of the so-called 'nanny state', where the state tells people how to live their lives. It is not that at all. Effective health communication is about ensuring the best possible opportunities for everyone to live healthy lives. By making full use of the evidence base, explaining to care home workers and their managers why personal protective equipment (PPE) was essential, helping people with learning disabilities to understand the concept of social distancing, reminding people to get a COVID test if they had symptoms, and then later, encouraging healthy people to be vaccinated against coronavirus, were all part of essential public health communications. All of these essential communications took place at every level, from local to national and, ideally, international.

b) Misinformation

Whereas the need for accurate, clear public information during the pandemic became crucial, there were many other sources of information circulating that were less helpful. Among the stories on social media were nuggets of truth as well as complete nonsense, presenting real difficulty for ordinary people to understand how best to conduct themselves to remain well, and to protect the most vulnerable in their communities.

Since this was a new disease with knowledge developing all the time, even the official advice available to the public changed frequently, which was disconcerting and contributed to limited trust of those in authority. That doubt was compounded by the conduct of people in positions of authority, including high profile politicians, some of whom, on occasion, flouted their own guidance or even laws. Whilst government policies to control the pandemic were announced and, during the course of the pandemic, changed, the extent to which these policies were actually implemented varied.

One important aspect affecting the success of communication of public health measures is the trust of ordinary people in those people or authorities who introduce them: if there is little trust, the measures are much more likely to fail due to lack of engagement or even outright rejection by the public. The parties involving cabinet ministers taking place in contravention of pandemic lockdown legislation are clear examples. Several senior politicians, advisors and staff members, were found to have broken one or more of the pandemic laws. These breaches resulted in some being convicted of mostly minor offences, while others resigned from ministerial office.

When members of parliament were suspected of continuing to mix socially during lockdown in this so-called 'Partygate scandal',[4] – the public, understandably, questioned why the rules should apply to them when their leaders appeared to be immune. Such lack of trust in England, in particular, may be contrasted with the situation and culture in other countries, such as Sweden and Japan, where trust in leaders was such that public health guidance was followed by the general population in some instances without the need for legislation.

Some politicians may also have been faced with conflicting interests, whether financial, personal or political. Politicians, unlike public health professionals, do not have a comparable ethical code and it is for individuals to decide how best to communicate with the public. They can be held to account, however, for their conduct through parliamentary – and where necessary, criminal justice – processes. In some cases, honesty gave way to self-interest.

As a result, it became very difficult during the pandemic to get messages from public health specialists taken seriously when high profile people were ignoring those messages.[5]

II) RESEARCH AND OTHER RELATED (MIS)EFFORTS

a) Official research

The virus responsible for the COVID pandemic was first identified and sequenced in January 2020 (in China). There followed a worldwide flurry of research activity to understand better this new organism that was causing global misery and how it might be tackled, by what are described by pharmaceutical (that is drugs and vaccines) and non-pharmaceutical (that is public health) interventions. There was a diversion of funds from other important areas of medical research in order to prioritise this, resulting in great opportunities for scientists working on research relevant to the pandemic, while research in those areas whose funds were diverted away suffered and, in some cases, continue to do so years later. This type of rationing did not have a high public profile during the pandemic, but the diversion of funds towards COVID-19, whilst rational and arguably essential, is likely to have longer term consequences for our understanding of some other diseases and their effective treatment.

b) Other suggestions of what might help

Alongside the research effort came an avalanche of ideas and suggestions from around the world about how best to treat patients who contracted COVID-19. Faced with a disease that was causing so many deaths, doctors wanted to try anything that might be effective. There were thousands of small-scale experiments of different treatments, most of which had no scientific rigour (meaning that the findings could not be relied upon) and some treatments carried additional risks for patients. Readers may recall, for example, the advice of then President Trump that people should consume disinfectant! Others recommended repurposing of old pharmaceuticals, such as the anti-worm drug Ivermectin, for which there was no evidence of its value in treating COVID-19 and, despite its popularity in some African countries during the pandemic, no benefit was ever proved. The pandemic became what many people working in public health and in clinical practice described as an 'evidence-free' zone, with, partly in desperation, the use around the world of a variety of medications and interventions that had no real value, in a sort of modern-day quackery. No doubt some purveyors of such so-called 'cures' made commercial gains as a result. Others may have thought they were doing some good.

III) CONTROL MEASURES

Public health measures are central to management of a pandemic. In the UK as in most other countries, ordinary people were told how to behave to reduce the risk of transmission (spread).

a) Lockdowns

On 23 March 2020, the Prime Minister, Boris Johnson, announced the first lockdown, which meant that people were required to remain in their own homes except when taking daily exercise. Apart from essential services like food shops, hospitals and public transport, most businesses were closed, along with schools. The latter went online with exceptions made for those children considered socially to be the most vulnerable. People who were known to have impaired immune systems were labelled as 'medically vulnerable' and the most vulnerable were advised – introducing the term 'shielding' – not to leave their homes, with arrangements made for food and medication to be delivered to them, in an attempt to minimise their exposure to the disease.

Lockdowns – where people's movements outside of their own homes were substantially restricted, usually by law– were a common public health measure, aimed at reducing the opportunity for the virus to spread. Whilst there is evidence that lockdowns can help to restrict spread of virus and, therefore, the number of people getting infected, seriously ill or even dying as a result of infection, lockdown policies resulted in many unintended adverse consequences. These affected children in particular, as a result, for example, of schools being closed affecting educational achievement as well as meals not being provided, loss of social contact and friendships, and social care services not accessing children at risk from domestic violence. Lockdown also had an impact on the economy, with much of the leisure, commercial and hospitality sectors closed. Whilst lockdown appears an effective intervention to tackle a pandemic, the total impacts of such policies went far beyond the pandemic itself.

The example of lockdown shows how a narrow approach to public health could aim to tackle infectious disease in isolation, while a more rounded or holistic approach would take into account the likely diverse – including some long-term – consequences beyond the infectious disease itself, all of which impact on the health and wellbeing of the population.

During 2020 and beyond, we saw many countries imposing lockdowns by law, such as across the UK, whilst a few comparable nations, notably Sweden, did not impose lockdown, but encouraged sensible social distancing behaviour while allowing some aspects of society – shops, businesses, restaurants – to remain open. Reviews are ongoing as to the wisdom of the variety of approaches employed. In a few countries, however, where the prevailing culture suggests that people routinely demonstrate trust in their national leadership, we have evidence that virus transmission was controlled without strict mandatory lockdown.

b) Face coverings

Policy concerning the wearing of face coverings also varied greatly between countries and in the same country over time. The evidence of effectiveness for non-surgical grade masks remains limited, but most countries introduced a policy of face coverings for the general public as part of social distancing measures at some time during the pandemic.

c) Fiscal help

Although not strictly a public health measure, the UK's central fiscal response is worthy of mention, since government funding was made available for employers to continue to pay workers during lockdown while they were not permitted to go to work, via a system described as 'furlough'. Such centrally funded, usually national, schemes provided wage subsidy or support. The funding allowed the lowest paid in society to maintain household income during the most difficult period of the pandemic. While comparable schemes were introduced in several countries, they were active for different durations. There were some high-income countries that did not introduce a furlough scheme at all, but which kept their economies 'open' throughout the pandemic. The best-known of these was probably Sweden, but Taiwan, Uruguay and Iceland similarly maintained their economies and a greater sense of normality.

IV) LACK OF PREPAREDNESS

A very high priority in the management of communicable diseases is preparation – readiness to respond effectively in the event of a major outbreak, epidemic or pandemic. Preparedness takes the form of ensuring that effective arrangements are in place for identifying cases:

- surveillance, testing, tracing, quarantining, and for isolating and caring safely for people who are confirmed to be infected;
- stockpiling of essentials such as PPE,[6] to ensure that sectors outside health are prepared – such as Education, Food, Treasury and
- have coordinated international preparations, via International Health Regulations (IHR)[7].

In the UK, we were not well prepared. Although a full review had been commissioned and its report published in the UK after the 2009 influenza pandemic,[8] many of its recommendations had not been implemented in the UK, although they had been adopted in some other countries, notably in the Far East.

V) MITIGATING MEASURES

Once an epidemic starts to take hold, the response has to shift from containment to mitigation (limiting the harm or damage). Sadly, during the Coronavirus pandemic, it took just a few weeks to reach this stage in many countries including the UK.

a) Social distancing

Public health measures included terms that, back in 2020, were new to most people, but they rapidly became well-known additions to the nation's vocabulary, and everyone suddenly knew about public health! First there was social distancing, meaning that people were expected to stand a few metres apart to reduce the risk of virus transmission from one person to another. Exactly what is the optimal distance apart remains elusive, but the government settled on two metres. In June 2020, the two-metre guidance was diluted, largely because of the economic burden, so that some workplaces could function with only one metre distancing. This was accompanied by additional mitigation measures including use of screens,[9] although people were reminded to maintain two metres wherever possible.

b) Handwashing

Another measure was washing hands, which we were exhorted to do after handling or touching anyone or indeed *anything* that might be infected, with the introduction, new to many people, of the concept of '*fomites*', or inanimate objects that might carry and transmit the virus. Later, the evidence indicated that fomites were but a minor source of infection, nevertheless the advice to wash hands and to do so adequately with soap, not just a cursory rinse, was sound. In the absence of soap and water, the use of hand sanitiser was recommended wherever we might touch an infected person or surface. Sales, as a result, soared. Suddenly, everyone walked about with sanitiser and even some alcohol distilleries were converted for production of sanitiser (with interesting odours reflecting their source) to help meet demand.

VI) THE IMPORTANCE OF VACCINE DEVELOPMENT

One crucial turning point in the evolution of the pandemic was the development of effective vaccines. Earlier, we mentioned the UK's investment in focussed research during the pandemic. A major part of this, which entailed impressive international collaborations, was vaccine development. Vaccination is one of the most effective preventive interventions that public health can offer. The development of new vaccines demanded the urgent, often international, collaborative efforts of experts from many disciplines. This resulted in the most rapid creation and trials of vaccines ever seen, including new technology that had never previously resulted in vaccine creation. The world's first mRNA vaccine was developed by a group led in the UK.

All the new vaccines licensed for use in the UK, wherever they were manufactured, were first subject to strict safety trials just like any new pharmaceutical products, followed by ongoing post-marketing surveillance, which in some cases led to restrictions of use among certain population groups. Some readers will have been volunteers on UK vaccine trials, without whom the vaccines would not have been released for wider use. Licensing was fast-tracked under emergency arrangements, so that the most vulnerable people in society and those who cared for them, could access the vaccine with minimum delay.[10]

At the local level in the UK, Directors of Public Health and their teams working in local authorities, were frequently central to ensuring safe and effective rollout, although the priority groups for immunisation were set out nationally, and online appointment systems were also centrally organised. Priorities for vaccination included initially the most vulnerable adults and frontline healthcare staff. Once evidence emerged that contracting COVID-19 in pregnancy was particularly hazardous and that the vaccine was safe in pregnancy, pregnant women were also prioritised. Later, children were included. Since 2021, the vaccination programme has been set on an annual basis, based upon the balance between costs to the public purse and likelihood of benefit. In 2024, for the first time, the vaccine was made available for private purchase by individuals – over the age of 12 years and outside priority groups eligible for NHS vaccination – who wanted the added assurance of immunisation.[11]

The success of vaccine development programmes, run by multidisciplinary teams on a global scale, and their subsequent national and international rollout were crucial in bringing the pandemic under control. It is estimated that, worldwide, over 14 million lives were saved.[12]

VII) OPPORTUNITIES FOR COMMERCIAL GAIN

Throughout the pandemic, there was no shortage of opportunities for commercial gain. Take, for example, the shortages of hand sanitiser early in 2020, when shopkeepers raised the price several-fold. Then came the bigger commercial players, who, in a seller's market, supplied PPE at high prices often to international buyers, whose own countries had failed to stockpile sufficient quantities for their own citizens.

Among vaccine manufacturers there were differences between those who decided to donate to a global vaccine pool, COVAX, which supplied vaccine to low-income countries, those who made their vaccine not-for-profit, and those who sold their product to the highest bidder. In the UK, when Brexit[13] was only just behind us, we watched with interest as our national vaccine procurement achieved what was reportedly a satisfactory and affordable supply, while UK media typically carried stories that suggested that countries within the European Union seemed to struggle for longer to reach consensus on procurement policy.

4. REFLECTIONS POST PANDEMIC

I) CULTURAL FACTORS

Cultural factors were crucial, for example in the case of masks. Countries where it was already common practice for people to wear a face covering when they had a cold or cough were very well prepared for that habit to be expected of them during the pandemic. Around the world, the requirement to wear a face covering varied hugely, both over time and in different environments. Whilst it might have been a widespread norm in a hospital or other healthcare environment, at different times during the pandemic face coverings were also mandated for travel on public transport, in taxis, walking outdoors, inside shops and even in restaurants while one was not actually eating.

II) COULD PUBLIC HEALTH SPECIALISTS HAVE OFFERED MORE BY WAY OF SOLUTIONS?

In any complex situation such as a pandemic, public health expertise is able to bring together objectively and impartially a multitude of important contributions, for example:

- identifying and describing the best available evidence of what works in managing serious outbreaks of communicable disease;
- understanding of the importance of essential processes including disease surveillance, contact tracing and testing;
- providing leadership to influence or manage particular actions;
- knowing how best to get complicated and often sensitive scenarios across to politicians, and
- knowing how to communicate health messages to the public most effectively to generate trust and compliance whilst avoiding panic.

This expertise involves having, and using, technical knowledge and skills as well as transferable or generic skills found in several occupations. Rarely do we find all of them together in one profession: public health.

To be effective, those working in public health had to display honesty and diplomacy as well as being articulate and confident in what they said or wrote. Specifically in the context of this pandemic they had to be able to remind the public that they were still learning, so that advice might have to change over time. Changing advice reflected both learning and uncertainty, which were difficult for the public to accept, when they wanted solid, authoritative expertise. Maintaining trust while being honest with the public was very challenging, but ethically imperative.

Depending on what access they had to a) accurate and complete information and b) the views of key decision makers (usually politicians), public health specialists were variably able or empowered to contribute to solutions. That applied at any level, whether local, regional, national or international.

At the local level, using their knowledge of their locality and population, the DsPH and their teams could advise, for instance, about how best to make testing facilities, then later vaccination centres, most accessible to the general public and minimise potential or actual inequalities. They could also help to monitor the progress of the pandemic through data sharing, which was not always straightforward due to data protection legislation.

Ensuring that local NHS and social care staff had access to adequate and suitable PPE was something that public health colleagues would recommend but, apart from using their voice in meetings, might not always be in a position to influence.

Likewise, at regional or national level, evidence-based interventions to address the pandemic with least adverse consequences would be recommended by public health experts, if they were fully informed and had access to decision makers. Sadly, the reality appears to have been that, at least early in the pandemic, public health leaders, particularly local DsPH, were not always included in communications that might have enabled them to offer sound advice for the benefit of their population.

Academic public health experts were very active in undertaking research, establishing the evidence base and in teaching other experts and the public alike about the pandemic. The London School of Hygiene and Tropical Medicine (LSHTM) developed rapidly and launched early in 2020 a university-standard, self-directed learning module (a MOOC: 'Massive Open Online Course') about this pandemic that was made widely available to all at no cost to students or other users. This, and other initiatives across the education sector, accelerated the worldwide development and roll out of online education, which became so important during the pandemic and subsequently.

The emergence and identification of inequalities

During 2020, differences in the way communities were affected by the pandemic were noticed, with clear inequalities emerging. An early example was the observation that the great majority of doctors who died while working during the pandemic were of Black and other minority ethnic backgrounds, many of them doctors who had come to the UK specifically to work in the NHS.[14]

At the clinical coalface, even where there was access to PPE, it was discovered that high grade protective masks had been developed to fit male faces and not female, and that males with facial hair were also disadvantaged in terms of fit. These might seem like minor details, but for frontline staff facing an unknown and lethal foe in their critically ill patients they amounted to significant inequalities.

From early in the pandemic, it was observed that some groups in the general population were hit hardest by COVID-19 and not all of these groups were anticipated from the experience of previous pandemics. During the first wave of the pandemic, people from some minority ethnic communities were more seriously affected than the population as a whole. After exploration of the data, it was concluded that living in multigenerational, often crowded households was behind much of the increased risk in older people from minority groups rather than ethnicity per se.

It was also observed that adults with learning disabilities were more likely to contract COVID-19 and to die from it than the general population. Whilst there is some evidence that some people with learning disabilities may have a suppressed (that is, less effective) immune system, an important reason for this observation was likely to be the great difficulty for some people to adhere to social distancing guidance and use of public health interventions such as hand washing.

Next, it was noticed that many people with type 2 diabetes became seriously ill or died following infection with COVID-19, again disproportionately compared with the general population of the same age. Reasons for this ranged from molecular level debate about differences in carbohydrate metabolism to the population level observation that, on average, people with type 2 diabetes were more likely to be overweight or obese than the population as a whole and were also more likely to have other medical conditions (known as comorbidities). People who were overweight or obese were more likely, therefore, to suffer poorer outcomes from COVID-19 than others. It was also established, however, that people with type 1 diabetes, who were more commonly of normal body weight, were even more likely to become seriously ill if infected with COVID-19. During the first wave of the pandemic in 2020, about a quarter of patients admitted to hospital because of COVID-19 had diabetes.[15]

Older people were particularly badly affected by the pandemic, with large numbers becoming seriously ill or dying. The existence of other underlying medical conditions played a part as did the natural wane in effectiveness of our immune systems as we aged. Added to the increased inherent risk was the risk brought by carers and others coming to visit older people, whether in a work or social context. People living in care homes were particularly badly hit by the pandemic. The lack of PPE and training for staff caring for these vulnerable people became apparent. This was compounded by patients being discharged from hospital into care homes while still infected with the coronavirus, thus likely contributing to its further spread.

5. THE PRESENT POSITION WORLDWIDE

The WHO declared an end to COVID-19 as a global health emergency (although not an end to it as a global threat) on 5 May 2023.[16] The coronavirus that caused the COVID-19 pandemic is now endemic[17] in most countries of the world and causes ongoing outbreaks of infection. The existence of effective vaccines has helped humanity live alongside this virus, although its constant ability to mutate means that it cannot be viewed as a benign feature in any society.

The end of the pandemic was not the end of the story, however. In March 2023, 1.9 million people across the UK (2.9% of the population) were still suffering the after-effects of COVID-19, known as long COVID or post-COVID syndrome. The most common symptom reported was fatigue followed by difficulty in concentrating, muscle ache and shortness of breath.[18] Long COVID was initially noted to be most common amongst people with pre-existing medical conditions, the elderly and those from poorer communities.

There have also been other health and social consequences to the pandemic. These included a widening of health inequalities as the impacts were felt most among the most vulnerable in society.

In terms of health, it has been observed that there is increased risk of people developing type 1 diabetes following COVID infection, a phenomenon also seen after some other viral illnesses. It appears to occur in people who already have subclinical type 1 diabetes, meaning they are predisposed to having clinical diabetes. The full condition is triggered by viral infection.

The pandemic has had a wider impact on the mental health of certain groups in the population, especially young people, disabled people and those in poorer communities. The periodic lockdowns, reduced social interaction, worries about access to health care and about finance all contributed. For those advised to 'shield' because of a vulnerability, isolation and loneliness became additional problems.

An international study on the effects of school closures during the pandemic on adolescent wellbeing found these impacted children's health and nutrition, their safety, education and employability, affecting particularly the most vulnerable and children in poorer communities.[19]

6. IN CONCLUSION

It has been estimated that during 2020 and 2021 there were nearly 15 million excess deaths associated with the COVID-19 pandemic in the population worldwide.[20] In England, in 2021 nine million cases were recorded and 78,128 deaths.[21] According to the WHO the future is not reassuring and the global risk assessment associated with COVID-19 remains high.[22] Nations have to be aware of, and be prepared for, the ongoing risk, as well as that posed by other organisms, some of which have yet to emerge.

What was special about this pandemic?

- A new virus;
- Speed of international spread;
- The first pandemic caused by a coronavirus;
- Unexpected risk factors for poor outcomes:

- Worldwide emergence of variants;
- High proportion of asymptomatic, infectious cases;
- Impact on non-COVID-19 healthcare;
- Unintended consequences of mitigation measures (eg lockdown);
- A pandemic in the age of rapid communications and social media;
- Long COVID…Post-COVID syndrome, and
- Inequalities.

The COVID-19 pandemic is a story of our time, but is just one episode in the continuing war between man and communicable diseases.

NOTES

1 Surveillance, prevention, outbreak control, case-finding, protective measures.

2 An epidemic refers to a sudden increase in the number of cases of a disease above what is usually expected. A pandemic refers to an epidemic that has spread over several countries or continents, usually affecting a large number of people. The cause of a pandemic might be a new (novel) organism.

3 King's Fund 2021. Directors of Public Health and the Covid-19 Pandemic. See: https://www.kingsfund.org.uk/insight-and-analysis/reports/directors-public-health-covid-19-pandemic

4 Numerous examples, including the infamous 'Partygate' scandal: https://www.bbc.co.uk/news/uk-politics-59952395

5 Rather like when doctors stopped smoking back in the 1960s, many other people followed their example, but the voices and actions of a cabinet minister, who happened to be a smoker and another in whose constituency sat the country's biggest cigarette manufacturer, probably contributed to delay in tobacco control legislation for years.

6 Personal protective equipment – essential for healthcare workers likely to be exposed to infected patients: note that some equipment was suitable only for males, leaving female staff exposed, while others were unsuitable for men with facial hair.

7 https://www.who.int/health-topics/international-health-regulations#tab=tab_1

8 Review conducted by Dame Deirdre Hine, 2010. https://assets.publishing.service.gov.uk/media/5a7975f1ed915d0422068a10/the2009influenzapandemic-review.pdf

9 https://www.gov.uk/government/publications/review-of-two-metre-social-distancing-guidance/review-of-two-metre-social-distancing-guidance
10 How have Covid-19 vaccines been developed so fast? See: https://www.immunology.org/public-information/vaccine-resources/covid-19/covid-19-vaccine-infographics/speed-of-development
11 This is a source of inequalities, since only people who can afford to pay or who wish to use their savings to purchase vaccine are able to make this choice and to benefit, leaving the rest of the unprioritized population without the protection provided by the vaccine.
12 'Lives Saved by COVID-19 Vaccines', *Journal of Paediatrics and Child Health*, 58(11): 2129, 20 September 2022: 10.1111/jpc.16213. https://pmc.ncbi.nlm.nih.gov/articles/PMC9537923/
13 Brexit was the process by which the UK left the European Union; it commenced in January 2020 and ended in December 2020.
14 https://www.bmj.com/covid-memorial
15 Of patients with diabetes admitted to hospital because of COVID, those with type 1 diabetes fared worse than those with type 2. This most probably reflects a major difference between type 1 and type 2 diabetes, with only type 1 being a disease of the immune system. High blood sugar was also associated with poor outcomes and people with type 1 diabetes often have higher blood glucose levels than those with type 2. https://www.cebm.ox.ac.uk/news/views/coronavirus-and-diabetes-the-different-risks-for-people-with-type-1-and-type-2
16 https://news.un.org/en/story/2023/05/1136367#:~:text=WHO%20chief%20declares%20end%20to%20COVID%2D19%20as%20a%20global%20health%20emergency,-5%20May%202023&text=The%20head%20of%20the%20UN,no%20longer%20a%20global%20threat
17 Always present in the population.
18 https://commonslibrary.parliament.uk/research-briefings/cbp-9112/
19 Gray, N.J. et al., 'Multiple Impacts on Adolescent Well-Being During COVID-19 School Closures: Insights From Professionals for Future Policy Using a Conceptual Framework', *Journal of Adolescent Health*, 77(3): 524–31. https://www.jahonline.org/article/S1054-139X(25)00156-9/fulltext
20 The difference between the number of deaths that occurred and the number expected in absence of the pandemic based on data from earlier years. https://www.un.org/en/desa/149-million-excess-deaths-associated-covid-19-pandemic-2020-and-2021

21 https://www.gov.uk/government/publications/covid-19-reported-sars-cov-2-deaths-in-england/covid-19-confirmed-deaths-in-england-to-31-december-2021-report

22 https://www.who.int/publications/m/item/covid-19-global-risk-assessment

FURTHER READING

UK COVID-19 Inquiry: https://covid19.public-inquiry.uk/

8

BODYWEIGHT

1. INTRODUCTION

This case study will consider body weight, in particular overweight and obesity, as a public health issue. Human bodies are not designed to be fat and there are serious health consequences of being overweight that continue to emerge. We shall look at why, in the twenty first century, such a large proportion of the world's population is overweight or obese and what can or should be done to address this important threat to human health.

2. WHAT IS THE PUBLIC HEALTH PROBLEM?

Obesity is a state of abnormal, unhealthy weight for any species, including humans. For millennia, we have known about the size and shape of mankind, which has evolved substantially over time. There have been increases in height and muscle mass, which mean that modern man is overall larger than his ancient forbears. This has been associated with steadily improving nutrition. But in recent times, that has changed, and we have seen an alteration in average weight over a few decades, accompanied by increases in stored body fat.

Unhealthy weight is a public health problem because being overweight is associated with many risks to health which, when scaled up to population level, affect the prevalence of certain chronic diseases, demand for medical and surgical treatments, and cause reduction in life expectancy.

Obesity is associated with increased risk of several types of cancer, type 2 diabetes, cardiovascular disease (many types of heart disease and stroke), high blood pressure, asthma and arthritis and

DOI: 10.4324/9781003779902-14

some types of mental ill health. In addition to the needs for healthcare, this huge and preventable burden of ill health means that people have greater need for sickness absence from work, affecting a nation's economy.

We can also note that provision has to be made for a population that is, on average, bigger than the generation before it, which is why, for instance, stadium seats and airline seats have become larger, even though most people might not have noticed. Whilst our focus will be chiefly on public health interventions, within healthcare provision there have been changes made to accommodate heavier patients, to which we shall return later in this chapter.

3. DEFINING OBESITY AND HEALTHY WEIGHT

Body weight is a sensitive issue and the definitions of being overweight, obesity and healthy weight in both adults and children are often viewed as a difficult area for discussion. It is, however, also essential to identify what we mean when we discuss these topics, particularly if we want members of the public to engage with their own health and if we intend to measure the impact of interventions that are aimed at tackling unhealthy weight as a public health issue.

For decades, healthy and unhealthy weight in adults have been defined by a measure called body mass index (BMI). BMI is a ratio of height and weight, calculated by dividing weight in kilograms by height in metres squared (BMI = kg/m^2). It is a valuable screening tool, but at the individual level it can be criticised, because if you are very muscular you may find your BMI in the less healthy range. BMI can also be problematic during pregnancy, although knowing that a person is overweight or obese at the start of their pregnancy is helpful in planning their care.

In adults, the standard categories for BMI are:

Healthy weight: 18.5 – 24.9
Overweight: 25 – 29.9
Obese: 30 – 39.9
Severely obese (sometimes described as morbidly obese): 40 or more
Underweight: 18.49 or less

Importantly, however, it has been discovered that people from some ethnic groups – including those from Asian, Chinese, Middle Eastern, Black African or African Caribbean backgrounds – are more susceptible to the adverse effects of obesity at lower BMIs than White populations. Thresholds, therefore, have been revised to show the BMIs at which those groups are more likely to encounter adverse health impacts. This does not mean that individuals are 'fatter', but that their metabolism seems to be more sensitive to being overweight and obese than people of White ethnicity. This is a complex area still under scientific scrutiny, but it means that people from these groups, and their medical advisers, should be aware of a higher risk to their health at lower BMIs, with the following advice from the NHS:

Overweight: BMI 23 – 27.4
Obese: BMI 27.5 or above

Today, additional measures are often used to decide if someone is overweight or obese. The use of waist circumference or waist-to-hip ratio may be superior to BMI for identifying people with central[1] obesity, who are now recognised to be at greatest risk of severe obesity-related ill health.

According to the NHS, at present, at least one in every four – or 25% – of UK adults are obese. A far greater percentage are overweight. A Report published on behalf of the Westminster Government in February 2025[2] reported that over two thirds of people in England aged 35 and over are overweight or obese. Furthermore, between 1995 and 2022 the proportion of adults in England who are obese *doubled*. As the global obesity pandemic grows, so too does the proportion of people who are obese or overweight.

4. HEALTHY WEIGHT IN CHILDREN

It is important to know that, on its own, BMI is an unhelpful indicator in children, whose weight has to be considered in the context of both age and sex. There are published charts showing children's healthy weights for both sexes (using sex assigned at birth). However, these have been criticised for being based on measurements of British children a few decades ago, since when the ethnic and racial mix of children in the UK has changed and, with that, their typical build and body composition. A 'one size fits all' approach is increasingly difficult to justify and reliable replacement charts to reflect the diversity of the UK population are being developed.

In England, about one in five – that's 22.1% – of 10–11 year old children (in School Year 6) were classified as obese and a further 13.8% overweight.[3]

5. REDEFINING HEALTHY AND UNHEALTHY WEIGHT?

Since the prevalence of overweight and obesity has been rising in recent decades, there have been occasional calls to redefine the terms for adults and children. In public health, however, we are concerned that redefining them to create new 'norms' would suggest that what was unhealthy is no longer the case, which would be misleading and potentially very harmful. As it is, some adult clothes manufacturers and retailers have altered clothes sizes over the years so that the consumer believes they are a smaller size than their measurements suggest or, certainly, than in their parents' generation.

For children's clothes, a wider range of sizes for the same age is often offered, to allow for different body shapes, which, while a great way to get clothes that fit better, helps to give reassurance to parents buying them that their child's body shape for clothes – which might be described positively using terms like 'super skinny' or 'plus fit'[4] – is quite unrelated to their health and wellbeing. Conversely, it is important to avoid stigmatising children or their parents who are overweight. Positive branding is understandable and also good for sales.

Increasingly, we see influencers and celebrities who are overweight or obese and who portray a positive image to their fans. The notion of 'body positivity' is impactful, particularly among young people, to remove stigma associated with appearance, which is important. However, there is a sensitive balance between the importance of removing stigma, whilst encouraging healthy living in terms of eating, drinking and physical activity and how they interact and relate to our body shape and weight.

Much of the argument for redefining and changing descriptors is about dealing with stigma. Sadly, overweight and obesity remain issues surrounded by stigma. It seems to be a very difficult balance to achieve an awareness of the importance to mankind of healthy weight, while not stigmatising or blaming those among us who are not.

6. UNDERWEIGHT

This case study is about obesity and overweight and their impact on the population's health, but it would be remiss to omit reference to underweight, which is itself a risk to health. Whole communities can be affected by inadequate nutrition because of failed harvests or other agricultural mishaps, conflict, natural disaster or disease. Any of these may lead to famine or even to starvation. At an individual level in both children and adults, eating disorders such as anorexia nervosa, where a person's food intake is insufficient for normal living, can lead to severe, chronic underweight and accompanying serious ill health or even death.

7. WHY HAS THE POPULATION BECOME MORE OBESE?

It is simple to say that if we eat more than we need, the excess calories (energy) we consume will be stored as fat and we are likely to get fatter. Let us look, therefore, at why the proportion of the UK population that is obese has increased so much in the past three decades, from 15% in the 1990s to 29% in 2022. Many other countries, including some more usually thought of as having starvation as a major public health challenge, have seen comparable increases in rates of obesity and it has become a global issue, which is sometimes described as a (non-communicable) pandemic.

It is complicated! We will not try to oversimplify it, but we will explain it. We can start with what food we eat and how much of it. During and following the Second World War, the diet of British people was largely dictated by rationing imposed by government, which was based on basic nutritional requirements. Later, a broader range of foodstuffs was more readily obtained, with much of it bought fresh and home cooked.

After a limited start in the 1950s with chains like Wimpy, there came the roll out across the UK of 'fast food' outlets in the 1970s of mainly US chains. There was suddenly easy access to food that was ready to eat and required no preparation or cooking skills or equipment, was generally affordable and, for the younger generations at least, fun to eat. The era of fast food was born.

Nutritionally, much fast food is relatively poor in nutrients, other than calories derived from fats and refined carbohydrates, and these ingredients make us want to eat more of them. They are made using technology now called ultra processing (UP) and we now know that ultra processed foods (UPF) can be addictive. So, we have now raised a few generations whose food preferences are very largely influenced by UPF. Indeed, in some places, there is very little other food available, with people living in 'food deserts', where it is impossible to buy fresh fruit, vegetables, raw fish or meat.

Unsurprisingly, the people most exposed to this diet of almost exclusively UPF are those who cannot afford to travel further to buy better food or who have neither cooking facilities nor skills, so that fast food or ready meals may be the only practical option to feed their hungry families.

We should also mention fizzy drinks. These had been around in the UK for several decades in the form of lemonade, cream soda and ginger beer but took off with the introduction, from the USA, of Coca-Cola©, then Pepsi© and other sugar-sweetened beverages, served in fast food outlets. The British public was introduced to these imported soft drinks, which rapidly became immensely popular and universally available for sale in retail stores and pubs as well as restaurants. Consumption of refined carbohydrates, especially sugars, in the typical British diet rose as a result of all these changes.

8. FOOD LABELLING

Although the UK has food labelling laws, it remains possible for labels to be difficult for people to read or to understand, and, in some cases, the presence of certain ingredients is played down by manufacturers. For example, although sugar might be listed as an ingredient, not all customers might notice the separate inclusion of fructose-glucose syrup (often called corn syrup in the US), dextrose or numerous other rather less obvious names for sugar. Then there are products, frequently marketed as healthy options, that have no *added* sugar, but are naturally high in sugar, such as some fruit juices.

Education plays its part, too. If you struggle to read, you are less likely to be able to take account of detailed food labelling. If you do not know that high sugar or fat content are a bad idea, then you would not limit your family's consumption of foods containing them. If you finished full-time education at GCSE or less, you are likely to be living on a lower-than-average income. We can see, therefore, the development of health inequalities, with unhealthy weight – overweight or obesity – being far more likely in people with lower family incomes than in the rest of society.

9. THE IMPORTANCE OF EXERCISE

What we eat is the biggest determinant of body weight, but how much energy we expend on being active is important, too. In a primitive world when people had to hunt for food for their families, they remained physically fit and not overweight. People ate to remain able to participate in whatever occupied them, whether that was hunting, foraging, building shelter, childbearing, childcare, washing, food preparation or fighting. The introduction in the twentieth century of motor vehicles, offices and factories, domestic appliances and multiple shops has led to a much more sedentary lifestyle. Many people, therefore, expend much less energy on a daily basis while consuming the same or greater quantities of food, the composition of which will also have changed substantially during the past 50 years. Inevitably, this has led to more people becoming overweight.

Among children, crucially, it has long been recognised that a child who is overweight or obese is much more likely than his or her peers of healthy weight to become an obese adult.

The reasons for people being physically inactive again point to social inequalities: poorly planned housing estates without safe play space or well-lit streets for walking or cycling, as well as being far from affordable good food shops, all contribute to making people less physically active. In the 1970s, the popularity of television was blamed for our increasingly sedentary lifestyle. Now we use screens, that we carry with us, for several hours a day, which is associated with even less time spent being active or outdoors.

10. INTERNATIONAL COMPARISONS

The social gradient in obesity is stark, with people living in the poorest areas much more likely to have unhealthy weight, along with their children, than people who live in more affluent neighbourhoods. This applies across the UK and internationally. Nations have expanded their waistlines at different rates. British people visiting Florida in the 1980s were astonished at the number of very large people they saw. The UK has since caught up, with now only a slightly smaller percentage of people who are obese than our American cousins. The UK now has the third highest rate of adult obesity in Europe, and the NHS spends more than £11billion per year on obesity related diseases.[5] Current government policy aims for a modest reduction in average calorie intake across the whole population, with essential participation by food industry players – agriculture, manufacturers, retailers and the leisure sector.

Across Europe, there is much variation between countries in shares of overweight people. As of 2022, for example, more than half the adult population in Europe was overweight or obese. It might come as a surprise to hear that males are more likely than females to be overweight or obese. In Latvia, for example, 56.7% of females were overweight or obese, while Italy had the lowest proportion at 31.3%. For males, the lowest proportion was 51.5% in France and the highest 69.4% in Slovakia, Malta and Croatia. In England, 71% of males and 62% of females were overweight or obese in 2022, with the trend continuing upwards.[6]

11. OBESITY AND THE COVID-19 PANDEMIC

Public health challenges hardly ever exist in isolation. Let us look at the relationship between obesity and the pandemic, for example. Unsurprisingly, it is not simple. But here are a few findings:

- People who were seriously overweight were, on average, more severely affected by COVID-19 than people of normal weight. This resulted in more admissions to hospital including to intensive care AND more deaths due to COVID-19 among obese people throughout the pandemic.

- Obesity was recognised as an independent risk factor for poor outcomes in COVID-19. That means that it was a risk in its own right, in addition to other risks, such as persons having type 2 diabetes or a severe learning disability.
- Obesity is linked with impaired immune function, which might help explain both why obese people seem more likely to contract COVID-19 and why they tend to suffer more seriously once they are infected.
- While the people most likely to become seriously ill from COVID-19 were the elderly, amongst obese people, they often became seriously unwell at a younger age.
- Obese people have been noted to be more likely than others to have post-COVID syndrome or long COVID.

12. OBESITY AND ALCOHOL

When it comes to obesity, the pandemic is not the only intersectional[7] public health issue. Take alcohol consumption, for example, which is a very long-established social habit in the UK. Recently, alcohol consumption has begun to reduce in the UK, with many younger adults not drinking alcohol at all but, of those people who do drink, some are drinking more heavily.

The reason for mentioning alcohol in this context is twofold: firstly, alcohol contains calories, which many of us do not think about when considering how much we drink and secondly, drinking alcohol boosts your appetite and people frequently eat a meal – often a fast-food take-away – with, or after, drinking alcohol. We are, therefore, more likely to consume more calories if we drink alcohol, unless we use alcohol as a meal-replacement, which, given its lack of nutritional value, is, in itself, a particularly unhealthy choice.

When offering personalised advice about achieving healthy weight, people should be reminded about the contribution of alcohol to their daily or weekly energy consumption, but it is rare to see this mentioned in advertisements for alcoholic drinks and neither contents nor calorie labelling is a current requirement in the UK.

Both alcohol and obesity are independent risk factors for several types of cancer, as well as other serious diseases, including cardiovascular disease (heart disease) and hypertension (high blood pressure).

13. WHAT ARE THE SOLUTIONS?

Being overweight or obese should be entirely preventable, or virtually so, with the exclusion of a tiny number of people who have medical disorders that directly affect their weight. The reality, as we all know by looking around us, is that tackling overweight and obesity is not easy at all.

Let us look at where solutions lie:

I) PREVENTION

Public health measures usually put prevention as the first choice, and it makes so much sense to prevent a problem rather than to try to tackle a tricky one once it has become established. Prevention will look different at local and national levels, and we shall explore these differences.

Prevention is sometimes regarded as simple. 'Prevention is better than cure' is an old adage, often true, but almost always much more complex and difficult to achieve than that simple phrase suggests. Obviously, everyone needs to eat to stay alive, so the solution is not a simple one about stopping doing something completely, as might be considered for other public health interventions, for example smoking, drinking alcohol, speeding or not wearing seatbelts.

First, what can be done locally?

Local councils and their public health teams

Local government is responsible for ensuring safe streets and for planning regulations that could encourage the provision of essential shops selling healthy food products to serve local communities and discourage excess fast-food outlets or their proximity to schools. Local councils, by commissioning affordable housing and approving all local residential developments, could ensure adequate, safe play space is always provided in these developments.

Local councils are responsible for providing playgrounds and parks, communal swimming pools and gyms, designed for people to access affordable places to be physically active. Town planners have a major role to play in public health, which has only become widely recognised in the past decade or so.

Local public health teams can engage with retailers to lead or support initiatives to promote healthy eating, for example, moving sweets from supermarket checkouts, offering free fruit to children instead, offering less attractive price promotions on sugar sweetened drinks, and aiming to influence other aspects of product placement and price that may result in healthier purchasing choices. Unless, or until, legislation is introduced, these initiatives are reliant on goodwill and a sound evidence-based approach with local businesses, many of which genuinely want to see their customers happy and healthy.

Schools

Schools are very important in tackling, ideally preventing, unhealthy weight. Their importance is about education as well as about being healthy places for children to spend much of their time. Despite education in schools including a requirement within the national curriculum to teach about health and to teach cooking, not all schools manage to deliver the latter. Schools are also required to provide opportunities for children of all ages to be physically active. School meals are expected to meet appropriate nutritional standards. All of these expectations are achieved with huge variation within a local authority area and around the country.

The National Child Measurement Programme

The National Child Measurement Programme (NCMP) in England started in 2006. It provides for height and weight measurement of every State schoolchild in Reception (age 4/5 years) and in year 6 (age 10/11) and gives feedback to parents. This has two functions, the first is to permit accurate monitoring of children's weight over time and to compare the weights of successive cohorts of children, the second is to provide information to parents with a view to empowering them to keep their families healthy. This latter aim has been challenging, with some parents reacting negatively to their child's results or the suggestion that it is their responsibility to address these. The sensitivities around how the programme relates to parents is ongoing and some schools have tried to help, for example, by involving parents in initiatives involving cooking or physical activity. It should be noted that children who are home-schooled as well as those attending private schools, are omitted from the NCMP and that there is no comparable programme in other countries of the UK. We do not yet know how effective the NCMP is in addressing childhood unhealthy weight, the impact of concerns about stigma, nor any disadvantage to those children who are omitted from the Programme.

What about national and international action?

Central government has levers for change that can influence major commercial and industrial players such as the leisure, food and agriculture sectors. If, for example, food manufacturers reduced the amount of refined sugar in everyday foods, we would see a drop in the whole population's sugar consumption. If North American farmers were to be incentivised to produce crops other than those for making corn syrup, we would see a drop in refined sugar consumption in the UK and globally. If bars and restaurants ensured preferential pricing for non-sugar sweetened drinks, again consumer habits would change. In fact, in the UK, we have seen a little of these types of changes, the best known being the 'sugar tax', whereby high sugar beverages are taxed at a higher rate than others. In practice, however, manufacturers or retailers often absorb the increased cost so that the price to the consumer is unaffected, limiting the impact of the tax on consumers.

In the UK, successive governments have been reluctant to introduce taxes or take other forms of regulatory action in relation to public health. The fear of being labelled a 'Nanny State' seems to concern politicians across the political spectrum, which means that we have little regulation and depend heavily on voluntary agreements with industry, with, once again, only limited impact on people's behaviour.

II) SOLUTIONS OTHER THAN PREVENTION

In public health, we frequently describe interventions as being upstream or downstream. An upstream intervention is usually preventive, put in place and implemented in advance of a problem arising. On the other hand, a downstream intervention picks up the pieces after the problem has become obvious and is often very serious.

We shall look at downstream interventions, because this is, at present, the dominant focus in the UK and many other relatively high-income countries. Some downstream interventions came from industry, recognising a commercial opportunity, while others were developed as part of government policy. Each of these examples will be considered through a public health lens in chronological order.

a) Diet foods

In the mid-twentieth century, it became fashionable for people, women in particular, to aspire to a very slim physique. This was not the physically fit shape that is preferred today, but thin, with a low body mass index (BMI). Women strived to achieve this chiefly by diet, and the market for diet foods took off. These took the form of meal substitutes, often drinks, with specified calorie values, so that the consumer would know precisely the number of calories they had consumed. Most were marketed to replace one meal per day, with ordinary healthy eating being promoted for the rest of the day. Some diet foods, however, were marketed as a complete replacement for normal meals. In addition, there were so-called healthy snacks, to replace 'unhealthy' standard snacks such as chocolate bars. These 'healthy' snacks usually had calorie values marked boldly on them. Although the calorie value was not always less than an equivalent standard snack or piece of fruit, the consumer was encouraged to view them as healthier.

b) Supportive meetings and clubs

Then came along organisations established solely to help people achieve their weight goals. Some were set up as clubs where people were encouraged to attend and meet regularly with others in the same position. Some were commercial entities or promoted specific diet foods manufactured or sponsored by the club owners. Commonly, participants paid a subscription, which was an incentive to succeed. In some cases, the NHS sponsored participation for people who were obese and on low incomes. These interventions used a behaviour change model, which was shown to be effective, although people who lost weight by also using meal replacements or other special food products, instead of eating healthily, tended to relapse and increase weight on stopping.

During the COVID-19 pandemic, when in-person meetings were impossible, these clubs went online: some have remained so.

In the UK, some of the most famous and successful of these organisations include Weightwatchers© and Slimming World©. In recent years, they have modernised, including physical activity as well as nutrition in their advice and support to members, and have developed apps for members to monitor their progress against goals.

From a public health perspective, this type of model can be effective if it is provided equitably, meaning it is accessible by anyone who is likely to benefit, rather than only those who can get to meetings or who have the app, and can afford to join and pay the subscriptions. In the absence of this equitable approach, health inequalities widen, as those of us who are affluent and mobile enough to join in may benefit, while others cannot. Health beliefs play a part, too. In many families, particularly in low-income areas, people are more inclined to believe that they, too, are destined to be overweight, because that is the pattern they see in their family. Breaking that trend and altering a firmly held belief based on lived experience is no mean feat.

c) Weight loss drugs in the twentieth century

Another phenomenon that became popular among some affluent people in the mid-twentieth century was the use of powerful drugs to lose weight. These were most often amphetamines, which were potentially dangerous and addictive. Some doctors prescribed these drugs or thyroxine privately for weight loss, which was hazardous and not licensed for this purpose. Ethical doctors would never advise such 'treatments' solely for weight loss in the 2020s.

d) Weight loss surgery

Surgical interventions for weight loss were first introduced in the 1950s in the USA, before becoming available internationally including in the UK. There are many procedures, but all are intended to reduce the capacity of the stomach, so that the person will then eat less at a single sitting. Some people achieve substantial weight loss following what is now known as bariatric surgery, others relapse. Counselling before surgery is important as is ongoing support afterwards. In the NHS, these surgical procedures are heavily rationed, with eligibility criteria including weight, evidence of previous attempted weight loss and existing underlying medical conditions. No surgery is without risk, and very obese patients are often at significantly increased risk, so fully informed consent is essential.

From a public health perspective, surgery for weight loss has a place, where sustained attempts at other means of losing weight have failed, and people have existing serious medical conditions that could benefit from weight loss.

Unfortunately, there is a story of inequalities here, too. Rationing in the NHS is inconsistent, so that people living in different areas have different chances of being eligible.[8] Although the social gradient in obesity and overweight is well-known, some evidence suggests that people living in poorest areas are least likely to access or to undergo bariatric surgery,[9] probably for complex reasons including the impact of rationing in their area or because people are less likely to seek help from their doctor.

The public health lens expects us to look at the needs of the population as a whole. Is it justifiable, then, to make available specialised surgery for weight loss, which arguably *should* be manageable by other, less invasive or less expensive interventions, when other patients may have to wait months for treatment for often serious, possibly life-threatening conditions? A core value of public health is the fair distribution of resources to achieve the best health for the whole population, and this takes us into a minefield of ethical debate.

e) Twenty first century weight loss drugs

Issues around human body weight have become steadily more medicalised. We risk losing the motivation for society to tackle by social interventions, access to plentiful supply of healthy, affordable food and encouragement of physical activity from childhood onwards.

In the twenty first century we have seen huge growth in development and marketing of drugs to treat obesity and overweight. This is in the context of a much greater proportion of the adult population being of unhealthy weight, indicating that, to date, population-wide preventive measures have largely failed.

While the people most likely to benefit from taking these drugs are those with serious underlying metabolic or cardiovascular diseases, these drugs have become to some parts of society 'lifestyle drugs', accessed by affluent people who simply wish to reduce their weight to optimise their healthy appearance and to maintain their ideal weight almost effortlessly.

A further problem is that they are sometimes accessed online by people with body dysmorphia leading to anorexia and used to reduce weight even further. Drugs such as GLP-1 receptor agonists, some of which were initially developed for treatment of type 2 diabetes, are used for weight loss. They are administered by regular injections, which many users can manage to do themselves. In the medium term, with drug company research investment, it is likely that these drugs will become available in tablet form, which is likely to make them even more accessible and more popular.

Whilst their availability and use in the NHS is limited by the application of evidence-based eligibility criteria, it is possible to purchase some GLP-1 receptor agonists online, where checks for eligibility – such as self-declaring one's weight or BMI – may not always be robust, even if the product itself is authentic. A separate risk of online purchases is that of fake drugs, which may have no therapeutic value and might even cause harm.

One of the unintended consequences of making these drugs readily accessible to affluent people in high-income countries is that this helps to contribute to an international shortage of some which have been repurposed from treatment of type 2 diabetes. Also of concern, as described by the WHO, is the increased falsification or sale of counterfeit drugs for the treatment of type 2 diabetes in some low-income countries.

It has been argued that a high proportion of the UK population could benefit from long term use of these drugs. This does not address the causes of being overweight, merely the result. That is not a public health approach and, while some of these concerns will be resolved in the years ahead, in 2025 the existing policy ignores a number of issues at both the population and individual level, including:

- the as yet unknown health risks of their long-term use among healthy adults (currently there appear to be short term cardiovascular health benefits);
- the probability of compliance with long term medication in the general population;
- the cost to the public purse, which could mean other NHS (or leisure or other publicly funded) services not being funded – that is, the 'opportunity cost' to the NHS of making weight loss drugs widely available;
- the permanent identification of human body weight as primarily a medical matter rather than an issue for society to address through other – upstream – means, and
- ignoring and therefore failing to address the major contributions of the huge multinational food and drinks industries to the pandemic of unhealthy weight.

14. IMPACT ON THE NHS OF OVERWEIGHT PATIENTS

I) SPECIAL EQUIPMENT

Earlier in this chapter we discussed the huge burden of ill health that is attributable to unhealthy body weight. We shall now look at its impact on healthcare provision over and above the additional burden of disease caused by obesity. These factors might not be obvious. For example, the NHS has invested in larger equipment, sometimes described as 'bariatric' equipment, for patients who are too large to be able to use regular equipment, such as standard hospital beds, imaging equipment (scanners, etc.).

While some patients might find it stigmatising to be referred to a unit that has these special pieces of equipment, prior to their introduction into the NHS, some routine investigations could not be offered at all to certain patients, so patient care fell below modern standards, and this was a clear example of inequality in access. In some cases, obese patients were referred, probably with substantial embarrassment, to undergo their investigations where larger equipment was available in some veterinary establishments.

II) RECOVERY FROM SURGERY

Then there is the possibility that the seriously obese patient may need longer to recuperate from surgery than a person who is not obese. Surgical procedures and healing can both take longer and carry more risk for the patient, meaning that length of stay in hospital for patients who are obese is likely to be longer on average than for other patients. There is also a greater risk of readmission to hospital for complications, including infection, following elective surgery.[10] The obese patient is more likely to need care in a high dependency (for example intensive care) environment post-operatively. However, there is also some evidence of an 'obesity paradox', whereby obese patients recover from elective surgery as well as or perhaps better than others: this counter-intuitive finding remains contentious and subject to further research.[11]

Many of these factors have been taken into account when guidance was introduced in the NHS, encouraging patients to reach an optimal state of personal health and wellbeing prior to elective surgery. Whilst this was intended as guidance for patients and the NHS, it has been used in many localities as a reason for introducing a policy that restricts seriously obese patients from accessing elective surgery until they have demonstrated weight loss.

Understandably, such policies are contentious and may be described as discriminating against obese patients. However, if there is sufficient evidence to show that outcomes of elective surgery are adversely affected by excess weight, it may make medical sense to ask obese patients to try to reduce their weight prior to surgery if that is possible. Ongoing research being conducted in the NHS hopes to identify whether weight loss prior to elective surgery can also help people to maintain a healthier weight afterwards.[12] The area is ethically very complex.[13]

Finally, it is worth recalling that several of the problems that patients with unhealthy weight encounter as they use elective healthcare – like slower healing after surgery, staying longer in a high dependency environment, risk of complications – apply also to patients who smoke. Ultimately, obesity costs the NHS billions of pounds every year, as does smoking, powerful examples for upstream interventions being so important.

15. AND SO, WHAT NEXT?

Overall, as a society, both nationally and internationally, we are at a sensitive point, where we could become increasingly dependent on long term drug use by the general population or we could choose to look upstream at the real causes of the obesity pandemic and tackle them. One might ask why we have reached this point?

We have known about the potential for primary prevention for several decades, but implementation would require sustained government commitment as well as the support of ordinary people. Across the political spectrum, governments are not strong on long term goals, quite the opposite. They are also reluctant to impose solutions on industry, when it is industry that is an essential source of taxes for government expenditure. And there are those who believe, sometimes above all, that a libertarian approach trumps any government interference.

When it comes to a chronic and worsening global and national problem like obesity, the public health approach seeks the best affordable long-term outcomes for the whole population. Affordable outcomes are most likely to come from prevention, which needs a sustained commitment and buy-in from many essential stakeholders. In the UK, attempts to achieve change by voluntary agreements with industry have, so far, achieved very limited success. Government action in the form of regulation can bring about change for the better, but governments have continued to be reluctant to impose them on industry or, indeed, the public. Where manufacturers have changed the formulation of foods voluntarily, for example, to reduce sugar or fat content, the changes are usually acceptable to consumers. Unless all the major food manufacturers, in particular, are on board with such changes, their impact is limited. Reformulation has costs, so that voluntary action is unlikely to be extensive without either regulation or loud public call for change and the latter is uncommon, especially in areas where most people lack detailed knowledge of the facts and most of us assume, incorrectly, that safe food is also healthy food.

If the government is to impose change which will have serious positive impact on the health of the whole population, its food policy would have to be robust, imposing on industry expectations of healthier formulations for many foods. Alongside this, we need education for the public to be better informed about ultra processed foods and for retailers to stock affordable, healthy options, including ending the 'food deserts' that exist in the poorest neighbourhoods of many towns and cities in the UK. We would need better access to facilities for everyone to be physically active, often the responsibility of local councils as described earlier.

Internationally, the World Health Organization supports initiatives for healthy eating and promotion of physical activity, but there are no sanctions for nations that ignore their guidance.

NOTES

1 Central obesity gives a rounded body shape that is most prominent around the midriff indicating that the internal organs lying below may be covered with fatty deposits.
2 https://researchbriefings.files.parliament.uk/documents/SN03336/SN03336.pdf
3 NHS Digital, National Child Measurement Programme 2022/3
4 Marks & Spencer 2025
5 https://www.gov.uk/government/news/healthy-food-revolution-to-tackle-obesity-epidemic
6 'EU Obesity and Overweight Statistics 2022'. https://ec.europa.eu/eurostat/statistics-explained/index.php?title=Overweight_and_obesity_-_BMI_statistics
7 Cross-cutting, found in combination with other factors.
8 https://www.bmj.com/content/386/bmj.q1950.short
9 https://academic.oup.com/bjs/article/110/Supplement_8/znad348.090/7428826
10 Elective surgery is used to describe admission to hospital (which might be for less than a full day or as an inpatient) for an operative procedure on a planned basis, not as an emergency. Across the UK, waiting lists and therefore waiting times, for elective surgery have grown substantially as a result of the COVID-19 pandemic, when services were focussed on the pandemic and not on the longstanding health needs of patients.
11 https://journals.lww.com/aosopen/fulltext/2024/12000/the_obesity_paradox_revisited__is_obesity_still_a.39.aspx#:~:text=The%20%E2%80%9Cobesity%20paradox%E2%80%9D%20suggests%20better,despite%20obesity's%20associated%20health%20risks
12 https://www.fundingawards.nihr.ac.uk/award/NIHR303187
13 https://ukpandemicethics.org/wp-content/uploads/2021/05/Government-Healthy-Weight-Strategies.pdf

SOURCES ACCESSED IN COMPILING THIS CHAPTER

BMJ, 'Food Industry Body Admits That Voluntary Agreements Lack Punch', *BMJ* 2016; 352:i1508. doi:https://doi.org/10.1136/bmj.i1508

Foresight, Government Office for Science. *Tackling Obesities: Future Choices—Project Report*, 2nd ed., 17 October 2007. www.gov.uk/government/publications/reducing-obesity-future-choices

UK Government Research Briefing on Obesity, 'Obesity Statistics', 10 February 2025. https://researchbriefings.files.parliament.uk/documents/SN03336/SN03336.pdf

WHO, 'Shortages Impacting Access to Glucagon-like Peptide 1 Receptor Agonist Products; Increasing the Potential for Falsified Versions', 29 January 2024. https://www.who.int/news/item/29-01-2024-shortages-impacting-access-to-glucagon-like-peptide-1-receptor-agonist-products--increasing-the-potential-for-falsified-versions

9

TOBACCO CONTROL – HALTING THE PANDEMIC

1. INTRODUCTION

Tobacco, and the smoking of cigarettes and related products, have been the scourge of public health for many decades. They continue to be one of the biggest threats to both public and individual health and tobacco control remains a global health priority. Access to cheaper, illegal imports is another issue that promotes smoking. Some of these problems, and potential solutions, will be explored later in the chapter.

I) HARMS TO HEALTH

Smoking, and exposure to environmental tobacco smoke ('passive smoking'), increase people's risk of developing a range of illnesses which can be fatal, or often cause irreversible long-term damage to health, including several cancers,[1] chronic respiratory diseases, stroke, dementia, peripheral vascular and cardiovascular disease.

Through passive smoking there are risks for non-smokers of developing smoking related diseases, especially lung cancer, cardiovascular and respiratory disease. Exposure to second-hand smoke is particularly harmful to children, exacerbating middle ear disease, asthma and allergies.

Despite the link between smoking and serious health issues having been established through epidemiological studies in the 1950s and 1960s,[2] influencing the majority of doctors at the time to quit smoking, it took many decades for restrictions on the sales and advertising of cigarettes to be imposed and disincentives introduced, such as high taxation and limitations on where cigarettes could be smoked.

DOI: 10.4324/9781003779902-15

II) HARMFUL TOXINS

The toxins in cigarettes[3] are harmful to health, while nicotine, a key component of tobacco, is addictive, triggering release of dopamine in the brain. This gives a pleasant sensation helping to relieve stress in the short-term. Nicotine addiction is one of the main barriers to stopping smoking and withdrawal symptoms can be hard to manage. There are numerous other barriers, including:

- smoking as an ingrained personal or social habit;
- misconceptions about the harms of nicotine which lead to reluctance to use nicotine replacement therapy;
- lack of effective support in quitting;
- social acceptability of smoking in certain communities;
- using smoking as a coping mechanism, particularly amongst people who are vulnerable, for example, because of homelessness or mental illness;
- the age of initiation, teenagers being especially vulnerable to addiction and, not least,
- persistence of the tobacco industry in marketing its products.

III) SMOKING A GLOBAL HEALTH ISSUE

The WHO estimates that tobacco kills more than 8 million people worldwide a year, 7 million from direct tobacco use and 1.3 million from non-smokers exposed to second hand smoke.[4] Today, 80% of the world's 1.3 billion tobacco users live in low- and middle-income countries (LMICs) where the burden of tobacco-related illness and death is now heaviest.

Tobacco use also contributes to poverty, as money for basic needs such as food, shelter and education is diverted to buying cigarettes. It also harms agriculture in poor areas where tobacco crops command greater reward than food crops.

The global prevalence of smoking may be declining (projected to be 15.4% of adults in 2025, down from 33.3% in 2000[5]) but progress is uneven and, as we shall see, inhibited in many parts of the world by tobacco company tactics. Figures from Cancer Research UK in July 2025 indicated that Britons still smoke 286 billion cigarettes a year. The way forward is helping smokers to quit whilst preventing people from taking up smoking in the first place, especially young people. A strong combination of local and national action is required.

2. HISTORY OF TOBACCO USE

I) ORIGINS

Tobacco originated as part of Native American culture where its leaves (smoked, sniffed and chewed) were used as a sacred medicinal plant in ceremonial cultural practices to promote well-being. From the late fifteenth century, sailors, returning from explorations in the Americas to various ports in Europe, took the practice of smoking with them in the form of pipe smoking in Northern Europe and cigar smoking in Southern Europe. From Europe, the practice spread gradually to the rest of the world. It did not become an item of mass consumption until the end of the seventeenth century, and, by the nineteenth century, it was an established practice across the world, whether through pipe smoking, snuff, tobacco chewing, cigars.

II) THE RISE OF WIDESPREAD CIGARETTE USE

Cigarettes were originally sold as an expensive handmade luxury item for the urban rich of Europe. The introduction of the rolling machine in the late nineteenth century brought inexpensive, mass-produced cigarettes widely to adult populations. This led to a decline in pipe smoking and tobacco chewing.

By 1950, half the adult population of industrialised countries smoked, and it was an acceptable form of social behaviour, popular across all social classes. In most western countries, smoking was predominantly a male activity until the middle of the twentieth century. This led to substantially higher rates in men than in women of lung cancer and coronary heart disease. This changed later in the century as smoking became ubiquitous among men and women.

III) THE DEVELOPMENT OF E-CIGARETTES

Electronic cigarettes (e-cigarettes or vapes) were first introduced in 2004 in China. Their use had spread to Europe and the USA by 2006. Although there has been much debate internationally, e-cigarettes are generally seen as a less harmful alternative to cigarettes because they do not normally contain all the toxins present in cigarettes. If used as an aid to quit smoking, they can help manage nicotine cravings and withdrawal symptoms. Experience has shown, however, that many users simply substitute e-cigarettes for standards cigarettes, leading to their long-term use and risk of relapse to tobacco smoking. Other people continue to smoke as well as using e-cigarettes so that any health benefit is very limited.

According to the WHO, the levels of some toxicants can be higher in some e-cigarettes and other emerging nicotine-containing products than in conventional cigarettes.[6] There is, moreover, little long-term data on whether these newer products are safer.

There are also concerns that non-smokers, including young people, are being targeted and encouraged to use them. This is in spite of the UK and several other countries having regulations that supposedly limit sales to adults. The inclusion of flavours and colours attractive to young consumers has been widely criticised. Vaping is potentially harmful to the developing lungs and brains of children and young people. In the UK, it is currently illegal to sell nicotine vaping products to anyone under 18, or for adults to buy them on their behalf. Single use vapes have been banned from sale in the UK since 1 June 2025 as an environmental protection measure, but some remain available via online sales. Their low price makes them attractive to children.

It is worth mentioning that most major vape manufacturers are owned by the major tobacco companies ('Big Tobacco'). This helps the industry continue to use the nicotine from tobacco crops and leaves open the real risk that, if vapes are withdrawn, a generation of nicotine-addicted people will return to smoking tobacco.

3. HISTORY OF TOBACCO CONTROL IN THE UK

I) EARLY EPIDEMIOLOGICAL STUDIES

The history of tobacco control in the UK has been painfully slow. Sir Richard Doll and Sir Austin Bradford Hill, British epidemiologists, first published their article postulating the link between smoking and lung cancer in the *British Medical Journal* (*BMJ*) in 1950.[7] They had been struck by the increase in the number of deaths from lung cancer, and, at first, thought it was due to air pollution. Their survey of hospital patients, however, indicated a link with smoking.

Following their 1950 publication they set up a long-term prospective (cohort) study to demonstrate the causal relationship between smoking habits and lung cancer beyond any reasonable doubt. Using the British Medical Register, they sent a questionnaire about smoking habits to doctors resident in the UK and collected over 34,000 questionnaires. This study soon showed that there was a strong association between smoking and lung cancer and, also, between smoking and cardiovascular disease. Although there were only 36 lung cancer deaths in the first 29 months of the study, after four years there were 200, almost all of them in heavy smokers. The incidence in non-smokers was negligible. Doll and Hill began publishing their results of this study in the *British Medical Journal* in 1954.[8]

Their studies were not at first taken seriously by the general public (although many doctors did stop smoking). After all, 80% of men in the UK at that time smoked. A 1962 Royal College of Physicians (RCP) report, *Smoking and Health*,[9] which recommended the government put restrictions on tobacco advertising and smoking in public places, tax cigarettes, and restrict the sale of cigarettes to children, was met with criticism and resistance.

II) GOVERNMENT ACTIONS

In the 1970s, half of the UK's adult population still smoked tobacco in one form or another. Rates dropped to a third by the 1990s, as the dangers became more widely apparent and restrictions started to be imposed. Since then, rates have continued to decline but at a slower rate (apart from during the COVID-19 pandemic when the decline stalled).[10]

The British government eventually *increased taxation* on cigarettes in 1965, and cigarettes were banned from being advertised on television. Smoking advertising was banned across all media from 2003. It was not until 2006/7, however, that *smoking was forbidden in indoor public places and the legal age of cigarette buying was raised to 18*. Since

1993, there has been a commitment by government to increase the duty (tax) paid on tobacco sales each year by at least 3%.

Mandatory plain packaging was introduced in the UK in 2015 for all tobacco products and a ban imposed on smoking in private vehicles if carrying children. Targets for reducing the prevalence of smoking in children, pregnant women and adults were introduced in 2017 as part of the *Tobacco Control Plan.*[11] New legislation, the Tobacco and Vapes Act, 2026, will forbid the purchase of tobacco by anyone born in the UK after 1 January 2009.

III) AMBITIONS TO BE SMOKE-FREE

Along with many countries world-wide, all four UK countries have the ambition to be smoke-free. In England in 2019, the government published a green paper *Advancing our Health Prevention in the 2020s*[12] which set the ambition for England to be smokefree by 2030, defined as adult smoking prevalence reduced to 5% or less. The government then commissioned Javed Khan, a former government minister, to review this ambition. He produced the *Khan Review: Making Smoking Obsolete* report in June 2022.[13] This advocated action needed to achieve the target which included increasing the age for the sale of tobacco by one year every year, promoting vaping as a smoking cessation tool, and improving quitting advice and support to smokers every time they had encounters with an NHS professional.

The current government is also funding more enforcement officers in local authority trading standards departments to help stop counterfeit or other illegal tobacco and vape products getting to neighbourhood shops, stop underage sales and tackle the crime groups organising them.

4. IMPACT OF SMOKING ON HEALTH IN THE UK

I) ILLNESS AND DEATH

Tobacco smoke remains the single biggest cause of illness, disability and preventable death in the UK, despite the numbers of smokers reducing. It has been estimated that over half a million hospital admissions in the UK in 2019/20 were directly attributable to smoking, the greatest number cancer-related, followed by respiratory diseases and circulatory diseases and, in 2019, caused nearly 80,000 deaths of adults aged 35 and over.[14] The most recent estimates from 2024 of the cost of smoking to the UK is reckoned to be £21 billion a year which includes costs of the burden on the health service and social care but also costs related to lost productivity, lost earnings, unemployment and early death.

Because of the 'lead' time between starting to smoke and becoming very ill, the falling prevalence of smoking lags years behind the burden of smoking-related diseases in society. Even after quitting, smokers carry an increased risk of many serious diseases, with the risk falling gradually over time, depending upon the number of years they were a smoker.

II) SMOKING IN PREGNANCY

Smoking in pregnancy has an impact on the baby, including increased risk of miscarriage, low birth weight, premature birth, still birth and sudden infant death syndrome (SIDS).[15] In England in 2023/4, 7.4% of women were recorded as smokers at the end of their pregnancy (down from 8.8% in 2022/3).[16] This is likely to be an underestimate because of the stigma associated with smoking during pregnancy and, also, that some women are thought to view smoking misguidedly as a way to restrict foetal growth and thus give birth more easily.

III) SMOKING AND WEIGHT

Another study of 83,000 adults in the UK found that smokers tended to eat less, and had less healthy eating habits, than non-smokers.[17] Nicotine can suppress appetite, and, for some people, smoking is used for weight loss. Stopping smoking was associated with weight gain.

IV) SMOKING AND HEALTH INEQUALITIES

Smoking status in twenty-first-century Britain is also associated with characteristics such as housing tenure, educational level and socio-economic status (approximate to income). It has been found that social renters are more likely to smoke, for example, than mortgage holders or those who own their property outright. People in a 'routine and manual' role are more likely to smoke than those in 'managerial and professional' occupations. Likewise, smoking is more common in those who have no educational qualifications compared with those with a degree or equivalent. This all amounts to a social gradient, with those at the lower end of the social spectrum much more likely to smoke than the most affluent in UK society.

Smoking is, therefore, associated with great health inequalities and is thought to account for half the difference in life expectancy (as much as four to five years) between the most and least well-off communities in England. It has been estimated that smokers spend an average of £2,000 disposable income a year that could be used for other essential or non-essential expenditure.

5. CURRENT SITUATION IN THE UK

I) CIGARETTE USE

The UK has still a way to go to be 'smoke-free' and reach a prevalence of 5% or less. From official statistics in the House of Commons Library, in the UK, in 2023, 11.9% of those aged 18 and over smoked, that is about 6 million people. Men are still more likely to smoke than women – 13.7% men compared with 10.1% women. Rates were highest in the 25–34 age group and lowest in those aged 65 and over. In addition, 9.8% of those aged 16 and over in 2023 in Great Britain were daily, or occasional users, of e-cigarettes.[18] Health surveys in Northern Ireland found young people started smoking because their friends did and most had started before the age of 18.

II) VAPING

In 2022, around 5.2% of people aged 16 and over in Great Britain were daily users of e-cigarettes and a further 3.5% occasional vapers, mainly in the 16–24 age group. Most of those using e-cigarettes were current or ex-smokers rather than people who had never smoked. Whereas smoking prevalence among school pupils is declining, use of e-cigarettes has increased. In 2021, less than 1% of 11–15 years olds reported regularly smoking. The ASH Smokefree Great Britain Youth Survey of 2024 of vaping among 11–17-year-olds reported, however, a prevalence of 7.2%. Fruit flavoured e-cigarettes made them more appealing, which reportedly increased experimentation among children.

III) CHEWING TOBACCO

Smokeless (chewing) tobacco is a form of tobacco used particularly by people from some minority ethnic groups in the UK, predominantly amongst South Asian men and women originating from Bangladesh, India and Pakistan. Continued use of these products is known to lead to increased risk of oral (mouth) and other health conditions including some cancers.

Cancer Research UK funded a smokeless tobacco study by York University across five boroughs in England which reported in 2021. In their study, the researchers found that products in half of the local shops surveyed were not legally permitted for sale in the UK. They also had packaging resembling confectionery. Plain packaging and graphic health warnings applicable to cigarettes do not apply to smokeless tobacco. They were also cheaper than cigarettes. The researchers called for better regulation,[19] which has been provided at least in part by the Tobacco and Vapes Act, 2026.

6. CURRENT UK SOLUTIONS FOR REDUCING TOBACCO USE

I) GOVERNMENT STRATEGY

The 2017 *Tobacco Control Plan for England* set out a map for the whole of the public health system to work together, nationally and locally, to bring about reduction in tobacco use. Local government should play its part in banning and monitoring of illicit sales, ensuring smokefree places, providing prevention and community-based smoking cessation services (although stop smoking services have been hit by funding cuts to local authorities and freezing of their Public Health Grant[20]).

The local NHS should treat tobacco dependency among patients who smoke. It must also ensure hospitals are smoke free. There was an expectation that GPs prescribe nicotine replacement therapy (NRT) or other stop smoking aids to patients. Pharmacies also should play a key role in providing stop smoking advice and support. Public health staff must work in collaboration with communities where smoking rates are highest.

II) NHS STOP SMOKING SERVICES

NHS Stop Smoking Services were established following the publication of the 1998 White Paper, *Smoking Kills*. They were initially piloted in one less well-off area of England in 1999 and rolled out across the UK from 2000. Of the more than 160,000 people receiving NHS 'support to quit smoking' in 2024, over half reported they were successful.[21] Various interventions, either alone or in combination, assist smoking cessation. These include brief advice from a health professional, behavioural support with therapies such as NRTs. There is some evidence that e-cigarettes may be more effective in aiding smoking cessation than NRTs, but questions remain regarding their safety and use in young people as described earlier.

III) RAISING THE COST OF CIGARETTES AS A DETERRENT

Among people trying to quit smoking, evidence suggests that concern for health was slightly more important than cost. The high cost of smoking can, nevertheless, be a useful deterrent. Tobacco tax duties are levied on the purchase of cigarettes, hand-rolled tobacco, cigars and other forms of tobacco. The Office of Budget Responsibility estimated that tobacco duties alone would raise £8.1 billion in 2025–26.[22] The Association of Directors of Public Health in 2023 considered it would be more effective if the government revised the tobacco tax escalator so that it is 2% above average weekly earnings rather than the RPI (retail price index).[23]

IV) PUBLIC HEALTH CAMPAIGNING

Public health advocacy may be a useful tool. In the smoking arena, a leading campaigning body, Action on Smoking and Health (ASH), has had, and continues to have, a key role in striving to end the harm caused by smoking in our society. ASH was set up in1971 by the Royal College of Physicians as a lobbying organisation because academic reports on smoking had not alone brought about change. ASH has used mass media and, more recently, social media, to help create the conditions for a shift in attitude towards smoking. It has also carried out direct actions such as buying shares in tobacco companies then turning up and disrupting shareholders' Annual General Meetings (AGMs) to draw attention to the health harms. Each year, it makes well researched submissions to government and parliamentary committees, and commissions annual surveys and reports on the state of smoking in the UK.

7. INTERNATIONAL SITUATION

Although overall, there is a global decline in smoking, one fifth of adults in the world still smoke tobacco whereas smokeless tobacco (ST) products are consumed by up to 351 million individuals worldwide with more than two thirds based in South-East Asia.[24] There remain a number of countries where more than a third of the population smokes, mainly in South-East Asia, the Pacific islands, and parts of Eastern Europe. Globally, there are still large differences between men and women. More than one-third of men in the world smoke whereas less than one-in-ten women do.

Of the 1.3 billion people aged 15 and over, estimated by the WHO, to have smoked in 2025, 80% live in low-and-middle-income countries (LMICs).[25]. Rates of smoking in these places amongst men is still increasing. Tobacco control presents a particularly challenging problem in Africa where deaths attributable to tobacco are projected to double by 2030. Despite a relatively low overall prevalence of smoking (18% of adults smoke), some countries in Africa are experiencing an increasing rate in tobacco use due in part to the fast growth of population and an increase in consumer purchasing power. Of deaths among adults due to second hand smoke, two thirds were of women living and working with men who smoke.

Many of today's high-income countries (HICs) had much higher smoking rates in the past and have seen a large reduction since the end of the twentieth century. Cigarette smoking first saw a significant rise in the wealthier countries in the early twentieth century. It peaked from the mid-to-latter half of the twentieth century before entering into a steep decline in subsequent decades.

This timescale is important when looking at the trajectory of smoking practices in low- and middle-income countries where widespread smoking has been adopted later than in high-income countries. If the former are to avoid the catastrophic health consequences seen by richer countries, they must accelerate efforts to reduce tobacco consumption.

Global efforts for smoking cessation are hampered in many countries by the actions of major international tobacco companies ('Big Tobacco') who actively market their products in LMICs. This undermines efforts by governments to curb the harms of smoking and is explored later in this chapter.

8. EXAMPLE APPROACHES TO TACKLING THE EPIDEMIC INTERNATIONALLY

I) COLLABORATIVE CROSS-COUNTRY APPROACH

The WHO developed a Framework Convention on Tobacco Control (FCTC) to support countries aiming to minimise the health impacts of tobacco. It was the first attempt by the WHO to have a global public health treaty. Adopted in 2003, and in force from 2005, the FCTC encourages countries to work to a common framework of (non-binding) obligations, and provides guidelines to enable comprehensive tobacco control legislation, as well as help them resist the pressure of the tobacco industry.

Actions recommended include banning tobacco advertising, protecting others from exposure to tobacco smoke, regulation of cigarette packaging, labelling and contents of tobacco products, raising the price of cigarettes through taxation and instituting measures to combat smuggling. As of 2024, 183 countries covering 90% of the world's population, were parties to the framework. The extent to which countries implement the recommended actions, however, is very variable.

In 2007, the WHO introduced MPOWER to provide high impact guidance for tobacco control, to reinforce messages and support countries in implementing the FCTC. MPOWER stands for:

- Monitoring the use of tobacco;
- Protecting people from tobacco smoke;
- Offering help to quit tobacco;

- Warning about the dangers of tobacco;
- Enforcing bans on tobacco advertising, promotion and sponsorship and
- Raising taxes on tobacco.

In 2022, more than 5.6 billion people in 151 countries (71% of the world's population) were covered by at least one measure from the WHO's MPOWER technical package.[26] There is still much to do, however. Comprehensive smoking cessation services, free or at subsidised cost to users, are available to assist people to quit in only 32 countries.

For a recent World No Tobacco Day (31 May) in 2025, the WHO FCTC urged signatories to ban the ingredients used to increase product attractiveness and palatability, such as sweeteners and flavours, in an attempt to combat the tobacco industry's attempts to market harmful products especially to children and young people.[27]

II) A POTENTIALLY SUCCESSFUL STRATEGY – SWEDEN

A number of countries, as well as the UK, have smoke-free ambitions of a 5% prevalence rate including Ireland, New Zealand, Canada and Finland.

Sweden, however, in 2024 was the first country in the world to achieve it. It did this by a combination of tobacco control methods and strategies to reduce harm from smoking. Only 4.5% of Swedish-born adults over 16 now smoke compared with an average of 24% across Europe.[28] Rather than focusing on abstinence or prohibition, the Swedish strategy was to encourage safer alternatives to cigarettes – snus (a moist smokeless tobacco placed under the upper lip), vapes and tobacco-free pouches containing nicotine.

A wide range of nicotine products, safer than tobacco, were made legally and cheaply available, supported by advertising and public awareness campaigns. Smoke-free products were cheaper than cigarettes. The aim was to make it easier for people to make healthier choices. Sweden had also undertaken prevention work from the 1980s to reduce the availability of tobacco products and decrease the demand for, and social acceptance of, smoking cigarettes.

The public health impact is seen in cancer statistics lower than the EU average, and a lower tobacco-related mortality.[29] It should be noted that Sweden has, however, not quit nicotine even if it has quit cigarettes. Most of the alternatives promoted carry some health risks, even if not as severe as from conventional cigarettes.

III) STATE CONTROL – CHINA

China leads the world in tobacco consumption and production. China has the largest smoking population in the world at nearly 316 million adult smokers. This accounts for almost one-third of smokers and 40% of tobacco consumption in the world. Some 27.7% of the adult population smoke (smoking prevalence) with a marked gender imbalance amongst smokers – 52.1% men and only 2.7% of women are smokers. An estimated 70% of the Chinese population, or more than 740 million people, are regularly exposed to second-hand smoke at home or work and this is helping to drive a lung cancer 'epidemic'.[30] In China, over two million people per year are expected to die from tobacco-related causes by 2026 and this figure is rising.

In some countries, including China, tobacco companies are State owned. Limiting tobacco use can threaten government income as well as growers' income as the State regulates and controls tobacco production. In 2014 the industry contributed nearly 7% of total income to the State.

In 2012, the WHO produced a report, *The Bill China Cannot Afford: Health, Economic and Social Costs of China's Tobacco Epidemic*,[31] which recommended a national smoke-free law, and raising tobacco taxes. China was already a signatory to the WHO FCTC. From 2015, the strategy in China changed and the State started to impose restrictions on smoking. A ban on tobacco advertising in mass media, public places, public transport and outdoors was imposed, as well as specifically prohibiting tobacco advertising which targeted young people. In 2016, the State published the *Healthy China 2030 Programme* which aimed to reduce adult smoking rates to 20% by adopting FCTC strategies including tighter banning of tobacco advertising, raising the price of cigarettes and banning smoking in public places.

The State has also reduced the acreage available for growing tobacco and substituted this with food. China is the first country to have such a policy of crop substitution around tobacco.[32]

These measures are in addition to smoking cessation support services. As elsewhere, smoking rates are higher among those of lower socio-economic status and educational attainment. There is also an urban–country split in China, with smoking more established in rural communities.

To date, smoking rates in China have been gradually decreasing, but at 27% in 2025, there is still a way to go to if it is to achieve its targets.

IV) FIGHTING FOR COMPENSATION AND THROUGH THE COURTS – THE USA

Cigarette smoking remains the leading cause of preventable disease and death in the United States. Adult cigarette smoking rates are slowly declining, dropping to 10.8% in 2023 compared with 11.6% in 2022, according to results from the CDC's 2023 *National Health Interview Survey*. As elsewhere, too, there are differences in who smokes by race and ethnicity, level of income, level of education. It is estimated that cigarette smoking and exposure to second hand smoke kill more than 480,000 Americans each year. Cigarette smoking cost the United States more than $600 billion in 2018, including more than $240 billion in healthcare spending and nearly $372 billion in lost productivity.[33] Cigarettes with flavours other than menthol were banned by Federal law in 2009.

According to the American Lung Association's 23rd annual *State of Tobacco Control* report in 2025,[34] the tobacco industry is taking a more aggressive stance at State level, seeking industry-friendly legislation or trying to gain exemption or reduction in State excise taxes on heated tobacco products and cigars. Campaigners are fighting in many States and localities to restrict the sale of menthol cigarettes and other flavoured tobacco products, including flavoured e-cigarettes, with partial success to date.

ASH USA has also reported an increased interference by tobacco companies in US public health policymaking. It cited one example from South Carolina in 2023 when industry-backed legislation was introduced with the aim of restricting local governments from imposing additional regulations on tobacco products. One of the bill's proponents had received campaign contributions from a tobacco company.[35]

In late 2024 public health campaigners secured one victory when the US Supreme Court refused to hear a tobacco industry challenge to the imposition of graphic health warnings on cigarette packs and advertisements required by the Food and Drug Administration (FDA). These warnings were initially required by Congress in 2009 but were repeatedly delayed by tobacco industry legal challenges. Graphic warnings were due to be implemented from December 2025.[36]

What has marked out the US, however, are the campaigns to gain compensation from tobacco companies. In 1998, 52 state and territory attorneys general signed the Master Settlement Agreement (MSA) with the four largest tobacco companies in the US to settle dozens of state lawsuits brought to recover billions of dollars in healthcare costs associated with treating smoking-related illnesses.[37]

The 'Engle Progeny Litigation' is a suite of lawsuits against tobacco companies filed in Florida courts since 1994. The original class action lawsuit included a paediatrician called Howard Engle who sought compensation for injuries suffered because of the health effects of smoking and the addiction it causes. The 'Engle' plaintiffs sought $200 million in damages. The court cases relating to this have been ongoing ever since. At one stage in 2000, a jury issued punitive damages of $145 billion but this was later capped.[38]

There is also the ethical issue of research funded by tobacco companies in the US, whether it can be relied upon and how might it be used. The American company, Philip Morris International, for example, has set up its own research facility with a sizeable fund to contribute to 'medical research'.[39]

V) THE CHALLENGES LMICS FACE IN IMPLEMENTING TOBACCO CONTROL MEASURES

a) Increasing numbers of smokers

Of the 1.3 billion people aged 15 and over who smoke worldwide now, 80% live in LMICs. Tobacco growing and consumption is now concentrated in the developing world where the health economic and environmental burden is heaviest. According to ASH, there are fears that the number of smokers may continue to increase because of population growth, income growth, increased tobacco affordability and aggressive marketing and political lobbying.[40]

b) Targeted marketing by Big Tobacco of women and children

As traditional markets in North America and Western Europe declined due to anti-tobacco initiatives and changes in smoking culture, transnational tobacco companies have expanded their sphere of operation in LMICs in Africa, Asia and Latin America where tobacco controls are less rigorous.

Targeted marketing is a particular risk for women in LMICs who traditionally are less likely to smoke. ASH found that targeted marketing of women included creating more 'feminised' products with packs resembling lipsticks or perfume as well as ultra-thin cigarettes. According to the WHO, 13% of adolescent girls in Africa now use tobacco products.[41]

In 2019, ASH reported that the tobacco industry was targeting children in Sub-Saharan Africa offering them free cigarettes.[42] The majority of child deaths from second hand smoke occur in Africa and South-East Asia.

c) Adverse impact of tobacco farming

Almost all tobacco farming (90%) takes place in low-income countries (LICs). There is also an environmental impact as, apart from deforestation to make way for tobacco agriculture, tobacco farming and cigarette manufacturing use large amounts of energy and water. Farming tobacco is hazardous for both adult and child workers due to the nicotine absorbed from the leaves of tobacco plants.

d) Underhand tactics deployed by Big Tobacco to prevent tobacco control measures

The WHO acknowledged in 2012 that the tobacco industry actively aims to undermine efforts to implement tobacco control policies through, for example, exaggerating the economic importance of the industry, manipulating public opinion, discrediting scientific research about tobacco harms and intimidating governments through litigation.[43]

Tobacco companies can also make it harder for countries to implement tobacco-control measures. In 2007, in India, multinational tobacco companies, local bidi (a thin, hand-rolled cigarette) producers and smokeless tobacco companies joined forces successfully to delay the introduction of graphic health warning labels. Pictorial health warnings on all tobacco products were eventually implemented from 1 April 2016.[44]

A review, from 2012, by Lee et al., of transnational tobacco companies' practices in LMICs to block tobacco control policies, and promote tobacco use, found they used four main approaches:

- economic activity (investment and smuggling) to enter new markets;
- political activity (lobbying, offering voluntary self-regulating codes);
- deceptive activities (manipulating science and using third party allies to oppose smoke-free policies) and
- marketing and promotion (tailored to specific market environments).[45]

The multinational tobacco industry also has a history of employing legal challenges or threatening letters to intimidate African governments and tobacco control stakeholders, either to stall the adoption or implementation of tobacco control policies or to weaken them. Sometimes, third parties are used as intermediaries.[46]

Another tactic is for the industry to use corporate social responsibility (CSR) activities to build support for policy positions that favour tobacco interests and improve its reputation, for example donations to 'support' response efforts in Uganda and Zambia during the COVID-19 pandemic.[47]

In 2025, the WHO issued an information sheet[48] warning about the tactics used by Big Tobacco to promote their tobacco and nicotine products including misleading labelling, referring to their products as 'clean' and 'less harmful' and using social media platforms to appeal to younger people.

e) *Slow implementation of the* WHO FCTC

It is important to recognise that the WHO does not have powers to impose action to be taken by nations that are signatories to its

FCTC. Of the 54 countries in Africa, 51 had ratified the WHO FCTC by 2021. Few African countries, however, had met the standards of the individual FCTC articles with regard to implementation. Africa has generally lower rates of taxation, weaker smoke-free policies and fewer restrictions on tobacco advertising and sales than many other parts of the world.

Some countries, including Ethiopia, Nigeria, Côte d'Ivoire, Niger and Madagascar have made progress, however, in adopting smoke-free laws, graphic pack warnings and comprehensive bans on tobacco advertising, promotion and sponsorship. Some 13 African countries had banned smoking in public spaces by 2021 and 16 required cigarette manufacturers to print graphic health warnings on cigarette packs.[49]

f) Taxation of tobacco

Other effective ways governments can combat tobacco use, advocated by the WHO, are tobacco taxes. A 10% tax increase in tobacco prices is estimated to decrease tobacco consumption by 4% in HICs and 5% in LMICs.[50] This should be combined with efforts to curb the illicit trade in tobacco products and attempts by Big Tobacco at undermining price increases.

One challenge for African countries is the failure to have effective excise tax systems which means cigarettes are relatively cheap. Raising the price via taxation almost always results in a decline in smoking. In South Africa, however, the government's inability to ensure tax compliance among tobacco manufacturers has led to an increase in illicit trade which accounts for a third of the market.

g) Setting up stop smoking support services

Smokers from less well-off families are less likely to quit in the absence of support services. At the local level, more could be done to implement low-cost smoking cessation initiatives such as brief advice from healthcare professionals, automated supportive text (SMS) messages and cheap therapies. Where senior health care professionals are in short supply to undertake intensive support, as a pragmatic approach, lower-level health care workers could be trained to give brief advice and support as part of an overall strategy (as has been done, for example, successfully with TB and HIV/AIDs).[51]

9. IN SUMMARY

This chapter has examined the public health problem of tobacco, still a huge cause of premature death globally. Although solutions are known and methods to promote reduction in smoking habits well tested, cigarette smoking is still proving an almost intractable problem in some areas.

Public health experts have contributed to research, public health campaigners champion reduction methods, local public health teams advocate smoking cessation practices and healthier environments.

The definitive solution may lie, however, in the willingness of governments to take a lead in implementing effective tobacco control policies and, in some places, to stand up to the major tobacco companies.

NOTES

1 Smoking is known to cause 16 types of cancer in men and women. https://www.cancerresearchuk.org/about-cancer/causes-of-cancer/smoking-and-cancer.

2 Smoking is the cause of death for about half of all along-term smokers. Doll, R. et al., 'Mortality in Relation to Smoking: 50 Years Observation on Male British Doctors', BMJ, 328:1519, 24 June 2004.

3 Tar, carbon monoxide and toxic chemicals.

4 WHO June 2025. https://www.who.int/news-room/fact-sheets/detail/tobacco.

5 https://www.statista.com/statistics/937294/tobacco-smoking-prevalence-globally/.

6 WHO Information Sheet 30 May 2025. 'Manipulation and Marketing Strategies Used by Tobacco and Nicotine Industries to Promote their Products'. https://www.who.int/publications/m/item/information-sheet--manipulation-and-marketing-strategies-used-by-tobacco-and-nicotine-industries-to-promote-their-products.

7 Doll, R., Hill, A.B., 'Smoking and Carcinoma of the Lung: Preliminary Report'. BMJ, 2(4682): 739–748, 30 September 1950.

8 Doll, R. and Hill, A.B., 'The Mortality of Doctors in Relation to their Smoking Habits: A Preliminary Report', BMJ, 1(4877): 1451–55, 26 June 1954.

9 https://www.rcp.ac.uk/media/csihjru3/smoking-and-health-1962.pdf.
10 In England rates fell from 5% a year to 0.3% between April 2020 and August 2022. https://news.cancerresearchuk.org/2023/12/14/decline-in-smoking-rates-stalled-during-the-pandemic-new-study-reveals/.
11 https://www.gov.uk/government/publications/towards-a-smoke-free-generation-tobacco-control-plan-for-england.
12 https://www.gov.uk/government/consultations/advancing-our-health-prevention-in-the-2020s/advancing-our-health-prevention-in-the-2020s-consultation-document.
13 https://www.gov.uk/government/publications/the-khan-review-making-smoking-obsolete.
14 'Statistics on Smoking', November 2025; https://www.gov.uk/government/statistics/smoking-profile-november-2025-update/smoking-profile-statistical-commentary-november-2025.
15 In Wales, for example, 15% of pregnant women were found to smoke at first assessment. Welsh Government, 'Maternity and Birth Statistics: 2021'. https://www.gov.wales/maternity-and-birth-statistics-2021-html.
16 https://www.england.nhs.uk/2024/08/women-smoking-during-pregnancy-at-record-low-thanks-to-nhs-support/.
17 https://leicesterbrc.nihr.ac.uk/uk-study-in-over-80000-adults-finds-smokers-tend-to-eat-less-and-have-a-less-healthy-diet-than-non-smokers/.
18 'Statistics on Smoking', 30 July 2025. https://commonslibrary.parliament.uk/research-briefings/cbp-7648/.
19 https://www.york.ac.uk/news-and-events/news/2021/research/stronger-regulations-needed-for-smokeless-tobacco/.
20 Annual ring-fenced grant to local authorities from the Department of Health and Social Care to fund certain public health functions.
21 'Statistics on Local Stop Smoking Services in England April to December 2024', published 24 April 2025, https://digital.nhs.uk/data-and-information/publications/statistical/statistics-on-nhs-stop-smoking-services-in-england/april-2024-to-december-2024-q3.
22 Office for Budget Responsibility, March 2025. https://obr.uk/forecasts-in-depth/tax-by-tax-spend-by-spend/tobacco-duties/.
23 ADPH, 'What we Say About… Tobacco'. https://www.adph.org.uk/resources/policy-position-tobacco.

24 ASH March 2020, 'Evidence into Practice: Smokeless Tobacco Products', https://ash.org.uk/resources/view/evidence-into-practice-smokeless-tobacco-products.

25 https://www.who.int/news-room/fact-sheets/detail/tobacco, 25 June 2025. There is no standard definition of a 'developing country'. North America, Europe, Australia, New Zealand and Japan are generally considered to be 'developed'. LMICs tend to have poorer economies, higher rates of poverty and mortality and lower standards of living in relation to higher income countries.

26 'WHO Report on the Global Tobacco Epidemic', 2023. https://www.who.int/publications/i/item/9789240077164.

27 https://www.who.int/europe/news-room/events/item/2025/05/31/default-calendar/world-no-tobacco-day-2025--unmasking-the-appeal.

28 The figure is 5.35 if immigrants are included.

29 https://www.businesswire.com/news/home/20241113569960/en/BREAKING-NEWS-Swedes-First-in-World-to-Become-Smoke-Free-Its-a-Lesson-for-the-World-Says-Smoke-Free-Sweden.

30 In 2015 there were over 700,00 new lung cancer cases and 610,000 deaths. Parascandola, M. and Xiao, L., 'Tobacco and the Lung Cancer Epidemic in China', *Translational Lung Cancer Research*, (Suppl 1): S21–30, 8 May 2019.

31 https://www.who.int/publications/i/item/9789290617907.

32 Other countries will have crop substitutions for example for cannabis and poppies.

33 https://www.cdc.gov/tobacco/campaign/tips/resources/data/cigarette-smoking-in-united-states.html#:~:text=In%202022%2C%20an%20estimated%2011.6,every%20day%20or%20some%20days.

34 https://www.lung.org/research/sotc/key-findings.

35 https://ash.org/wp-content/uploads/2023/10/2023-U.S.-Tobacco-Industry-Interference-Index-Report.pdf.

36 https://www.fightcancer.org/releases/victory-public-health-us-supreme-court-refuses-hear-tobacco-industry%E2%80%99s-challenge-graphic#

37 https://www.naag.org/our-work/naag-center-for-tobacco-and-public-health/the-master-settlement-agreement/

38 https://www.publichealthlawcenter.org/sites/default/files/resources/tclc-fs-engle-progeny-2015.pdf.

39 https://www.pmi.com/who-we-are/our-views-and-standards/standards/scientific-research.

40 'ASH Fact Sheet: Tobacco and the Developing World', July 2019. https://ash.org.uk/uploads/Tobacco-Developing-World.pdf.
41 WHO Africa. https://www.afro.who.int/health-topics/tobacco-control.
42 ASH Fact Sheet: Tobacco and the Developing World', July 2019. https://ash.org.uk/uploads/Tobacco-Developing-World.pdf.
43 WHO Tobacco Industry Interference: A Global Brief, 31 May 2012; https://www.who.int/publications/i/item/WHO-NMH-TFI-12.1.
44 Hoe, C., Kennedy, R.D., Spires, M., Tamplin, S. and Cohen, J.E., 'Improving Implementation of Tobacco Control Policies in Low- and Middle-Income Countries: A Proposed Framework', *BMJ Global Health*, 4(6), 16 December 2019.
45 Lee, S., Ling, P.M. and Glantz, S.A., 'The Vector of the Tobacco Epidemic: Tobacco Industry Practices in Low and Middle-income Countries', *Cancer Causes Control*, 23(01):117–129, 28 February 2012. https://pmc.ncbi.nlm.nih.gov/articles/PMC3332051/.
46 One example of tobacco industry interference cited was British American Tobacco (BAT) sending a letter to the Minister of Trade in Uganda in 2020, to share inputs on the draft tobacco control regulations received from the said Minister's office. However, this document was the official custody of the Ministry or Health, meaning that an informant at the Ministry of Trade had provided the document to BAT. https://web.archive.org/web/20211007111617/https:/exposetobacco.org/country/uganda/.
47 'Tobacco Tactics', University of Bath, 1 February 2022. https://www.tobaccotactics.org/article/african-region/.
48 WHO 30 May 2025. https://www.who.int/publications/m/item/information-sheet--manipulation-and-marketing-strategies-used-by-tobacco-and-nicotine-industries-to-promote-their-products.
49 https://www.afro.who.int/health-topics/tobacco-control.
50 https://www.who.int/news-room/fact-sheets/detail/tobacco.
51 Peer, N. and Kengne, A-P., 'Tobacco Cessation in Low- and Middle-income Countries: Some Challenges and Opportunities', *Addiction*, 113(8): 1390–91, August 2018. https://pubmed.ncbi.nlm.nih.gov/29663631/.

SOURCES ACCESSED IN COMPILING THIS CHAPTER

WHO, 'Tobacco', 25 June 2025. https://www.who.int/news-room/fact-sheets/detail/tobacco.

WHO Framework Convention on Tobacco Control, 3 March 2021. https://fctc.who.int/who-fctc/overview/parties.

WHO Framework Convention on Tobacco Control, 30 May 2025, 'WHO FCTC Urges Parties to Prohibit Ingredients Used to Increase Product Attractiveness and Palatability'. https://fctc.who.int/newsroom/news/item/30-05-2025-who-fctc-urges-parties-to-prohibit-ingredients-used-to-increase-product-attractiveness-and-palatability.

GOVERNMENT

Department of Health, 'Health Survey (NI): Smoking in Northern Ireland 2010/11 to 2019/20', April 2022. https://www.health-ni.gov.uk/sites/default/files/publications/health/hsni-smoking-trends-19-20.pdf.

Department of Health, 'Ten Year Tobacco Control Strategy for Northern Ireland: Final Review', 25 September 2023. https://www.health-ni.gov.uk/publications/ten-year-tobacco-control-strategy-northern-ireland-final-review.

Department of Health and Social Care, 'Smoke-free Generation: Tobacco Control Plan for England', 18 July 2017. https://www.gov.uk/government/publications/towards-a-smoke-free-generation-tobacco-control-plan-for-england.

GOV.UK, 'Smoking Tobacco: Applying All Our Health', 4 July 2025a. https://www.gov.uk/government/publications/smoking-and-tobacco-applying-all-our-health/smoking-and-tobacco-applying-all-our-health.

GOV.UK, 'Historical Tobacco Duty Rates', 29 August 2025b. https://www.gov.uk/government/statistics/tobacco-bulletin/historical-tobacco-duty-rates.

GOV.UK Press Release, 'More Officers on Streets to Smoke out Illicit Tobacco and Vapes', 23 March 2025. www.gov.uk/government/news/more-officers-on-streets-to-smoke-out-illicit-tobacco-and-vapes.

Office for Health Improvement and Disparities, 'Nicotine Vaping in England: 2022 Evidence Update Main Findings, 29 September 2022. www.gov.uk/government/publications/nicotine-vaping-in-england-2022-evidence-update/nicotine-vaping-in-england-2022-evidence-update-main-findings#.

Office for National Statistics (ONS), 'Adult Smoking Habits in the UK: 2023', 1 October 2024. https://www.ons.gov.uk/peoplepopulationandcommunity/healthandsocialcare/healthandlifeexpectancies/bulletins/adultsmokinghabitsingreatbritain/2023.

UK Parliament, House of Commons Library, 'Tobacco and Vapes Bill 2024–25: Progress of the Bill', 14 February 2025. https://commonslibrary.parliament.uk/research-briefings/cbp-10193/.

UK Parliament, House of Commons Library, 'The Smokefree 2030 Ambition for England', 16 October 2023. Commonslibrary.parliament.uk/research-briefings/cbp-9655/.

ASH

ASH, 'Evidence into Practice: Smokeless Tobacco Products', March 2020a. https://ash.org.uk/resources/view/evidence-into-practice-smokeless-tobacco-products.

ASH, 'Our History'. Ash.org.uk/about/who-we-are/our-history

ASH, 'Second Hand Smoke', March 2020b. https://ash.org.uk/resources/view/secondhand-smoke.

ASH, 'Use of Vapes (E-cigarettes) among Young People in Great Britain', July 2025. https://ash.org.uk/resources/view/use-of-e-cigarettes-among-young-people-in-great-britain.

REPORTS

Association of Directors of Public Health, 'Policy Position: Tobacco', 2023. adph.org.uk/wp-content/uploads/2023/04/ADPH-Tobacco-Policy-Statement-2023-1.pdf.

Britannica, 'A Social and Cultural History of Smoking'. https://www.britannica.com/topic/smoking-tobacco/A-social-and-cultural-history-of-smoking

Campaign for Tobacco-Free Kids, 'States and Localities that Have Restricted the Sale of Flavoured Tobacco Products'. https://assets.tobaccofreekids.org/factsheets/0398.pdf.

CDC Tips from Former Smokers, n.d. 'Burden of Cigarette Use in the U.S.' https://www.cdc.gov/tobacco/campaign/tips/resources/data/cigarette-smoking-in-united-states.html#:~:text=In%202022%2C%20an%20estimated%2011.6,every%20day%20or%20some%20days.

Department of Health and Social Care, 'Fingertips: Public Health Profiles'. https://fingertips.phe.org.uk/profile/tobacco-control/supporting-information/smokingandinequalities.

Folkhalsomyndigheten (Public Health Agency of Sweden), 'Towards a Smoke-free Sweden'. https://www.folkhalsomyndigheten.se/the-pubic-health-agency-of-sweden/living-conditions-and-lifestyle/andtg/tobacc/towards-a-smoke-free-sweden/.

Royal College of Obstetrics and Gynaecology (RCOG), 'Smoking and Pregnancy', updated 2020. https://www.rcog.org.uk/for-the-public/browse-our-patient-information/smoking-and-pregnancy/.

Royal College of Physicians, *Passive Smoking and Children*, London, March 2010. https://shop.rcp.ac.uk/products/passive-smoking-and-children?variant=6634905477.

Our World in Data, 'Smoking', Hannah Ritchie and Max Rosen, Revision November 2023. https://ourworldindata.org.smoking.

World Innovative Sustainable Solutions (WINSS), 'How Sweden Made Smoking (Almost) History', Evelyne Hoffman, 25 March 2025. https://www.winssolutions.org/how-sweden-made-smoking-almost-history/.

ARTICLES AND BOOKS

Berridge, V., *Public Health: A Very Short Introduction*, OUP, 2016.

Dobbie, F., Hickock, R., Leonardi-Bee, J. et al., 'Evaluation Long-term Outcomes of NHS Stop Smoking Services (ELONS): A Prospective Cohort Study', *Health Technology Assessment*, 95(1): 1–156, November 2015.

Hannah, R., *In which countries do people smoke the most?* 2019, Published online at OurWorldinData.org. Retrieved from https://ourworldindata.org/which-countries-smoke-most.

Li, V.C. and Tang, S., 'China's New Road for Tobacco Control: Tobacco Crop Substitution', *American Journal of Public Health*, 108(10): 1316–1317, October 2018.

Marshall, A-M., Siffiqui, F. and Dogar, O., 'An Evidence-based Guide to Smoking Cessation Therapies', *Journal of Prescribing Practice*, 5(8), 2 August 2023.

McKee, M. and Krentel, A., Issues in Public Health: Challenges for the 21st Century, 3rd edition, 2022. https://www.mheducation.co.uk/issues-in-public-health-challenges-for-the-21st-century-9780335249152-emea-group.

10

THE FUTURE – OBSTACLES AND OPPORTUNITIES

1. INTRODUCTION

Public health is steeped in tradition – tackling outbreaks of communicable disease over many centuries for example – and, at the same time, striving to adopt new developments that might help societies to live healthier lives. The three previous chapters have illustrated how difficult it is to deal with late twentieth- and twenty-first-century public health problems. Looking to the future while continuing to learn from the past is important, interesting and complex.

In this chapter we shall explore continuing challenges, some of which we have touched on earlier in the book, as well as new challenges we think are going to become increasingly important in the coming decade or two. We will look at potential opportunities for change.

2. CONTINUING CHALLENGES

I) COMMUNICABLE DISEASE CONTROL: LOOKING TO THE FUTURE OF TRADITIONAL PUBLIC HEALTH

Communicable diseases, and ways to tackle them, are constantly changing. Just because we know how to control a disease does not mean that control systems are always in place where and when they are really needed. Emerging infections such as the coronavirus that caused the COVID-19 pandemic are unexpected phenomena. With development of big data, effective global surveillance and scientific interventions that work, the next pandemic, or the one after that, could be predicted and effective vaccines developed within weeks

DOI: 10.4324/9781003779902-16

or even days of the causal organism being identified. A major outbreak would then look very different if we had the organisational skills and political commitment to ensure that the UK – or perhaps every country – had optimal pandemic preparedness in place, as well as the knowledge and skills to control the outbreak effectively, before the organism caused huge numbers of deaths or wrought havoc with healthcare service provision.

Emerging and often challenging new diseases such as a novel coronavirus are just one part of the diversity of communicable diseases facing mankind and the animal kingdom. In many countries, particularly low-income countries, some communicable diseases caused by organisms that have been very well known to mankind for decades or even centuries, kill many thousands of people, many of them children, annually. Most of these deaths are preventable. The reason that people die is because the basic tools to control these diseases – including tuberculosis (TB) and malaria – are not accessible by most people living in countries where the disease is endemic.[1] This is an example of health inequalities on a global scale which is preventable through better international cooperation and aid.

II) COMMUNICATION

Technical know-how and financial aid are not, however, sufficient to meet public health challenges. What the population believes and trusts in health communication and messaging is just as important – their perception of risk, belief in scientific evidence and their ability to discern the truth from the huge amounts of information bombarding them every day, especially on social media. This was touched on in Chapter 7 in relation to the COVID-19 pandemic and will be explored in more detail here.

a) Information

Clear, accurate information that is accessible to everyone is obviously desirable. Unfortunately, information about health and disease is often complex and people do not always understand it. Sometimes people want to believe their own ideas are the right ones, even if the expert evidence tells them something else.

More troubling are the phenomena of *misinformation* and *disinformation*. Misinformation is the dissemination of inaccurate or simply incorrect information as if it were true. This can happen accidentally or intentionally. Disinformation, on the other hand, is always the result of an intentional act to mislead people by putting incorrect information in the public domain, usually via social media but also by other means. Disinformation is especially harmful, because it allows lies to spread among an unsuspecting public and can cause people to make decisions based on untrue assumptions.

One of the most egregious and harmful forms of disinformation in health communication concerns vaccines, where there is an abundance of authentic-looking but fictitious data and stories about the harmful effects of vaccines. In Part 2 we described the article published in *The Lancet* in 1998 by Andrew Wakefield and withdrawn only many years later. The damage that resulted was extensive and long-lasting because the article was widely cited in mass media at the time and later. Uptake of MMR vaccine plummeted, not only in the UK but around the world, and has never recovered fully. Equally worrying is that uptake of other vaccines has been affected by 'association', despite the lack of plausible evidence of serious harm.

More than 20 years later, when new vaccines were developed during the COVID-19 pandemic, a sizeable community of anti-vaxxers became a loud negative presence on social media, causing many people to doubt the safety of the new vaccines. This contributed to less-than-optimal uptake in some populations.

Vaccine hesitancy is a normal reaction to something we do not understand fully, to which a helpful response is further explanation from, and discourse with, trusted sources. Anti-vaxxers, on the other hand, are willing to oppose all use of vaccines on the basis of fraudulent, fabricated evidence. Some anti-vaxxers even contribute to racial tensions, for example, by accusing vaccine manufacturers or healthcare providers entirely falsely – including by using conspiracy theory – of targeting certain groups within the population by injecting harmful products into them.[2]

Ways to counter such disinformation are to ensure that people are as well informed as possible about these and other health issues via trusted sources of information. Public health experts are well placed to do this.

Members of the public will then feel empowered to make the right decisions for themselves and their children.

There is no such thing as an entirely safe medicinal product, but vaccines developed and licensed in western democracies are among the safest and most effective.

b) Communication of risk

We saw in Part 2 how a misleading article on the risk for women in taking the contraceptive pill in 1995 caused many women to stop taking it. Incorrect presentation in the media of risks to health is a continuing problem. For example, a very small increase in *absolute risk of* cancer as a result, say, of exposure to radiation, can be described as a huge increase in *relative risk*. If the *absolute risk* increases from one in a thousand to two in a thousand, that probably does not sound too bad, but if someone – an ambitious journalist, perhaps – wanted to present an exciting headline, they could say that the *relative risk* has doubled! And if the word 'relative' is omitted or poorly understood, that can rapidly cause panic among those who read or hear it.

We see this in the opposite direction, too, where the benefit of an intervention is downplayed by malign players, such as anti-vaxxers, while risk of harm might be exaggerated by applying risk data inappropriately.

Ensuring that a reliable assessment of risk is completed and published with minimum delay by a trusted source, such as the local director of public health, or the Chief Medical Officer, sets the record straight and stifles the panic that might otherwise set in. At local level the DPH often has a good working relationship with the media to enable publication of clear stories and avoidance of this type of headline, while nationally and increasingly in the age of social media, the very rapid speed of publication and dissemination means that the trusted voice of public health is more likely to be engaged in damage limitation.

III) ACCESS TO AFFORDABLE HEALTHCARE

On average, according to the World Bank, countries spend around 10% of gross domestic product (GDP) on health. In the UK, this figure sits at about 11%. In the USA the spend is 16.5% GDP, while in Sub-Saharan Africa it is typically about 5% GDP.[3] Importantly, spending more does not necessarily result in better health for the population, as is clear from the USA experience. Although, as we have already discussed earlier in the book, healthcare provision is just one of many determinants of health in the modern era, the great majority of people would agree it is important that everyone has fair access to healthcare when they need it.

As we have seen in Part 2, there are huge inequities in accessing healthcare, even within the UK where, in accordance with the aspirations of the founding fathers of the NHS, we have universal access to healthcare that is (mostly) free at the point of use. Many nations do not have universal access to healthcare, including some of those that spend most on healthcare, such as the USA.

Looking to the future, how might healthcare become accessible fairly to everyone in need, regardless of their ability to pay, their social status, literacy level or other relevant variables? The public health response to this question has been to explore options for the affordable provision of healthcare as well as consideration of better access to preventive interventions and to social care.

In a socialised health system, trying to balance preventive interventions with care or curative interventions has proved challenging, because, in general, people want to receive care for their illness here and now. They do not want to be told that they must wait because the healthcare budget is being spent on prevention of someone else's ill health. Ultimately, the government could spend more public funds on health, but that would require political commitment and taxpayer (voter) agreement, a situation that we have yet to see in the UK.

In the UK, the balance has yet to be achieved, though it is continuously being sought. Countries such as the USA, where there is not yet societal acceptance of universal access to healthcare, have a range of other barriers to prevention, including conflicts of interest among both those providing care and those large corporations responsible, at least in part, for causing ill health amongst the population (as in the sale of tobacco).

In the UK, the application of ethical considerations at both the individual and population levels is of central importance in striving for fairness. There is a principle of distributive justice by which public resources – in this case those of the NHS – are intended to be shared equitably among the population to meet its needs.

One practical aid to this is NICE, the National Institute for Health and Social Care Excellence. NICE was established in 1999 and charged with producing 'useful and usable guidance for the NHS and wider health and care system'. They 'help practitioners and commissioners get the best care to patients, fast, while ensuring value for the taxpayer'.[4] They do this by applying ethical and economic principles to whether or not a treatment should be made available in the NHS in England. NICE's deliberations and recommendations are highly valued, however, some difficult decisions still have to be made at operational level, which include what expensive treatments to fund or not to fund.

Although not perfect, the methodology used by NICE is aimed at fair distribution of scarce, or at least finite, NHS resources. In the UK, some patients are able to choose to seek treatment privately, in which case a drug that is approved for use for this condition by the Medicines and Healthcare products Regulatory Agency (MHRA), but not approved by NICE for use in the NHS, might be prescribed to an individual patient privately, often at great cost, and sometimes covered by private health insurance. While one patient may benefit in this scenario, other patients who do not have access to non-NHS treatment, are relatively disadvantaged, a source of health inequality.

Apart from costs of healthcare provision itself, other factors that make access to healthcare inequitable, as we have seen in Part 2, include physical distance or difficulty in reaching services by public transport, lack or cost of childcare, loss of earnings, ignorance of the importance of attending an appointment or a language barrier.

A public health approach identifies these and other factors likely to cause further harm to already disadvantaged communities and supports development of policies to address them. If such an approach prevails throughout the NHS in future, we could look forward to less, not more, inequity in access to essential healthcare. Sometimes quite simple interventions, such as a specialist tertiary[5] clinic being made available every few weeks in a peripheral town's small hospital as an outreach service, can make a big difference to access for local people.

IV) WAR AND CONFLICT

a) The public health problem

It is perhaps all too obvious that war, which is directly responsible for deaths, often very many deaths, among civilian and military populations, is bad for public health. Our future world is as unlikely as any other era to avoid war, so we are including conflict, of which war is a powerful part, as a continuing major public health concern.

War and lesser conflicts affect mortality, since there has not been a war that does not result in loss of life which is in excess of what would be expected in normal times. As well as deaths due to bombings and other weapons, people are harmed by failures of public amenities such as water supply, shops and access to incoming foodstuffs, and, in some instances, a complete or partial breakdown in civil society and in local and/or national government. Healthcare facilities may become inaccessible due to damage caused by war or as a result of enemy occupation. People who are injured through war, may well need inaccessible medical attention including surgery.

When local society becomes unsustainable, war causes mobility, with populations being displaced, usually temporarily, but sometimes in the long term, depending on the conflict's outcome in relation to the population concerned. Displaced populations may remain together to re-establish their community elsewhere, perhaps near their original homes, or they might be permanently displaced to another land, where existing local communities might be more or less welcoming.

In recent years the enduring and even intergenerational impacts of war on the mental wellbeing of non-combatants have begun to be recognised. Adults and children living through war have an increased risk of mental illness and unsurprisingly, suitable therapeutic interventions, in the form of medication or a range of psychological therapies, may not always be available.

b) How a public health approach can help

A public health approach would include consideration of all types of impacts, so that, even where prevention is sadly impossible, appropriate services can be put in place to mitigate and manage all types of health impacts on a population in a timely manner, which may mean over decades. Initially, a public health approach[6] comprises supporting and restoring access to basic healthcare services as local to where people are living as possible. More sophisticated health services may take longer to establish. Public health professionals will advise on priorities for the local population working in partnership with affected communities wherever possible. These will include maternity and paediatric services, as well as public health services, such as adequate nutrition, immunisation, malaria prevention interventions, clean water and hygiene facilities.

c) The scourges of knife and gun crime

Knife crime in the United Kingdom

Conflict on a more local level is also a public health problem. In the UK, we have a longstanding problem of knife crime, often, but not always associated with gangs, and frequently affecting young people. We have checks on some students upon entry to their school to ensure they are not carrying knives. Every year in England and Wales about 250 people are killed as a result of knife (or other sharp object, usually a broken bottle) crime, amounting to almost half of all murders.[7] In 2024/5 about 3,500 people were admitted to hospitals in England because of knife crime.

In recent years, elements of a public health approach have been introduced to prevent knife crime, through collaborative work between police, education, health and other statutory stakeholders. Efforts include regulation of knife sales, bans on certain types of knives in schools and on the street, amnesties and greater engagement of charities and local communities. Data show that knife crime is geographically variable, with the highest incidence in England in London, Manchester and the West Midlands. A sensitively targeted approach is often needed. For the first time in many years, knife crime statistics declined slightly in 2024, which might be a positive early sign. After a crime has been committed there are opportunities for prevention of repeat knife crime, through interventions involving probation and prison services. Public health has a long, but often poorly resourced history of working with criminal justice services on programmes aimed at rehabilitation of offenders and prevention of future crime.

Gun crime in the United States of America

In the USA, gun crime has long been recognised as a public health issue. In a country with a very relaxed approach, compared with many others, to the sale and ownership of firearms, it is relatively easy for people to access a gun. There is an ingrained culture of gun ownership, fuelled by a powerful gun lobby as well as strong resistance among much of the voting public to any legislation that would restrict that 'right' to own a firearm and to participate in legal hunting and shooting recreational activities.

Following the murders by two peers of 13 fellow pupils and one teacher, as well as injuries to many more, at Columbine High School in Colorado in 1999[8], attempts were made to tackle gun crime as a public health issue. Decades later, similar incidents continue to recur with accompanying loss of young lives. Intermittently, the issues of gun ownership are raised.

The US response to gun crime, however, has focused on what we would describe as the downstream tackling of crime through the criminal justice system rather than upstream prevention where the focus would be on reducing gun ownership and access to firearms. Until Federal government and the American electorate decide that gun ownership is less important than the lives wasted as a result of gun crime, it is difficult to be hopeful that the problem will be addressed.

3. NEW CHALLENGES

I) ARTIFICIAL INTELLIGENCE

It has long been recognised that new technologies, including the application of artificial intelligence (AI), must be planned responsibly, taking into account its potential for causing harm as well as good. AI, and its introduction into healthcare, is no different.

The pace at which AI is being developed, however, and made available to everyone is in marked contrast to the usual laborious and lengthy process of research and development in healthcare. New drugs and products for use in medical practice are normally subject to extensive trials and evaluation, which are themselves subject to ethical standards and break clauses should certain scenarios occur. The development of AI is happening with relatively little regulation or restriction. It is necessary to ensure that safeguards are in place in the event of malign actors becoming involved in AI development and rollout. Scaling up of AI to extend its reach is considered to be a major benefit of this technology. To do so safely and ethically would be vital principles from a public health perspective.

Some countries are further ahead than others in implementing AI in healthcare or in public health. Learning from their experiences is essential. It is in the USA that investment, development and use of AI in health care is currently most advanced.[9] While AI is already in use to improve administrative efficiency, support development of personalised healthcare and tools for robotic surgical intervention, for example, critical challenges include ensuring safe and ethical implementation of these innovations at scale. Kaiser Permanente is one of the United States' biggest integrated healthcare systems and has introduced some principles for safe roll out of AI:

Privacy
Reliability
Outcomes focussed
Transparency
Promote **E**quity
Design tools for **C**ustomers
Trust[10]

Since our focus is on public health, it is important to consider how AI might impact on the health of communities and populations, and even on professions, not just on individual patients.

The UK government announced a new Commission for introducing AI in the NHS in the autumn of 2025.[11] There is a view that the UK should be a world leader in this area. A trial of the use of AI to improve NHS efficiency in administrative tasks is reportedly looking promising.[12] Since screening is a population health intervention, it is also worth noting that in September 2025, the government announced a research programme using AI to roll out enhanced screening – initially breast screening – to begin in 2027.[13] Reliable, safe machine-generated screening could transform prevention in medical care and allow medical experts to use their time for activities requiring human intervention.

AI is a potentially powerful tool to aid health improvement by reaching diverse communities and individuals with important health messages. For example, some communities that have poor uptake of immunisation could benefit from tailored messaging. Competent prompting via AI could adjust the health messages to best suit particular communities far more efficiently than a person creating and repeatedly editing content. If that results in improved vaccine uptake, this, in turn, would represent real improvements in the public's health.

In summary, while embracing the effectiveness and efficiency that AI might bring, there is clearly a need for caution in the use of AI, since there is clearly the capacity to do harm as well as good, either intentionally or unintentionally as a result ultimately of human initiated actions. Harnessing AI as a tool for good in public health terms should be a key aim of public health research, policy and practice in the current era.

II) CLIMATE CHANGE

a) Introduction

Without action, climate change and its sequelae, could, later this century, become the world's most important public health issue.

Climate change refers to long-term shifts in average temperatures and weather patterns across the planet. The average temperature of the Earth's surface is now about 1.2° Centigrade warmer than it was in the late 1800s (before the Industrial Revolution). This is warmer than at any time in the last 100,000 years.

Human activities, primarily linked with the burning of fossil fuels such as coal, oil and gas after the Industrial Revolution, are largely responsible for the present era's temperature rise. These activities, seen in agriculture, transport, construction and the oil and gas industries, release what have come to be known as greenhouse gases – mainly carbon dioxide and methane – that trap the sun's heat, making the earth warmer leading to extreme weather events, including heatwaves, floods and wildfires.

Direct consequences of climate change are the immediate impacts from these extreme weather events, such as injury or displacement. Indirect consequences are the secondary effects from these events such as worsened air quality, health problems and lack of food and clean water as well as the potential for economic instability.

'Net zero' is the necessary point to stop global warming, thereby preventing the most devastating impacts of climate change by balancing the greenhouse gases released into the atmosphere with those removed. This balance would help keep global temperatures to no more than 1.5°Centigrade above pre-industrial levels set by countries at the Paris Agreement on Climate Change of 2015.[14] According to international consensus on contemporary research findings, achieving net zero would protect human health and preserve biodiversity. Achieving this requires, however, a significant shift away from fossil fuels to renewable energy, improvements in energy efficiency, and active removal of remaining carbon from the atmosphere.

A decade after the Paris agreement, progress is mixed, but 83% of the global economy now has a 'net zero' target. The USA is notably absent. The picture is mixed and complex, with some hopeful advancements in some areas, such as solar and wind energy, but major concerns in others, such as energy use on air conditioning as temperatures increase and, perhaps surprisingly, energy use on electric vehicles and on AI.[15]

The Paris Agreement of 2015 included a global goal to strengthen resilience and reduce vulnerability to climate change. Climate change affects the less well-off and least polluting countries disproportionately. They are also the countries least able to adapt.[16] In future, climate change may increase risk of conflict linked to scarcity of resources including water, mass displacement of people and migration. Addressing the health impacts of climate change requires collaboration and cooperation across countries.

The WHO leads the Alliance for Transformative Action on Climate and Health (ATACH). In May 2025, it produced it Draft Global Action Plan on Climate Change and Health focusing on the following areas – leadership, coordination and advocacy, evidence and monitoring, country-level action and capacity building.[17]

b) Climate change as a public health issue

Climate change inevitably has an enormous impact on the health of human populations. Heatwaves, for example, can cause dehydration and heatstroke and increase the frequency of stroke. Extreme heat, drought, wildfires and flooding harms agriculture which could lead to food shortage. Safe water supplies are already endangered by drought and floods. According to the WHO in 2023, between 2030 and 2050, climate change is expected to cause a quarter of a million more preventable deaths each year from undernutrition, malaria, diarrhoea and heat stress.[18]

Even in high-income countries such as the UK, the increasing occurrence both of heatwaves and cold winters are serious problems, where few properties are energy efficient and the proportion of older people who are most vulnerable to heat and cold, is high. The UK has had high and rising excess winter mortality for decades and now excess summer mortality is rising too. By the 2070s, it is estimated that the UK could suffer over 21,00 additional heat-related deaths each summer if there are no improvements to housing such as better insultation and more efficient energy use.[19]

In addition to increasingly hot, drier summers leading to poor domestic harvests and reduced reservoir levels, the UK's reliance on imported food from countries affected by floods, extreme heat, wildfires and droughts may lead to problems with food supply and quality here in the UK.

Climate change leads to widening health inequalities. The most vulnerable groups in society, such as older people, poorer people, people with serious medical conditions or disabilities, and children, bear the greatest risk. Low-income households are more likely to be in environments which are less resilient to climate change, in areas likely to flood, and which have less access to green space.[20] Disadvantaged groups have, therefore, greater exposure to the potential harms to health due to climate change, suffer more from the consequences, and are least able to recover from them.

c) How a public health approach can make a difference

Even if a reduction in carbon emissions were to bring the increase in temperature to 1.5 degrees Centigrade above pre-industrial levels, societies must still develop more climate resilient and environmentally sustainable health systems to protect ourselves, our communities, and our environment. The solutions lie in mitigation and adaptation:

Mitigation refers to actions taken to reduce or prevent the emission of greenhouse gases into the atmosphere, thereby limiting the extent of future climate change.

Adaptation refers to adjusting to actual or expected climate change effects, making changes in our ways of life to lessen the negative impacts of climate change.

The public health approach, and accompanying expertise, could make a valuable contribution to both. Leadership, partnership, influence, advocacy, data, evidence, evaluation, communication will all come into play.

Central to public health intervention is ensuring services and policy makers focus on reducing the health inequalities stemming from climate change. Public health professionals can propose evidence-based ways to prevent, or minimise, further deterioration in inequalities and promote adaptation to the 'new' environment where appropriate.

Below are examples of how those working in public health could help, working with local communities, local and national bodies.

National policy

Strategies that rely solely on individual initiatives are unlikely to help communities prepare for, and adapt to, the vicissitudes of climate change. They may *increase* health inequalities, because uptake of measures, especially if they have a monetary or other cost to individuals or families, will vary depending on income and social status.

Policy and action at the national level are crucial, such as measures to ensure food safety and robust building regulations. Extreme weather events pose a new challenge to the UK which is more suited to a temperate climate. Preparations need to be in place to mobilise emergency services via early warnings and specific national plans. One example is the Adverse Weather Plan (2025/26) for England[21] which included strategies for vulnerable groups, such as older people living in care homes, and assisted in the development of more joined-up plans in different service delivery organisations. The UK Health Security Agency (UKHSA) has an Extreme Events and Health Protection (EEHP) team responding to adverse weather events such as storms and floods with the aim of mitigating health impacts.[22]

National policy, in order to reach the UK goal of reducing carbon emissions to Net Zero by 2050, will, among other actions, need to 'decarbonise'[23] the energy sector, phasing out coal and investing in renewable energy sources, 'decarbonise' transport by phasing out petrol and diesel cars, ensure new buildings are carbon neutral and assist adaptations to older housing. This is a huge agenda. The UK Climate Change Act of 2008[24] requires the government to undertake five-yearly assessment of climate risks and produce a National Adaptation Plan to respond to any identified risks including health and wellbeing.

Those working in public health can help inform policy makers by providing evidence of what works or does not work for different communities, including a focus on those groups most at risk.

Local services

Local Authorities are well placed to work with their local communities to limit the worst aspects of climate change. The impact of climate change will be felt most by low-income families whose housing is likely to be of lower quality, cold in winter and hot in summer. These households have to spend a disproportionate amount of money on energy, meaning less available for food and other essentials, a situation described as *fuel poverty*.[25]

The Director of Public Health and public health teams working in, or with, local authorities use tools such as health needs assessments, health impact assessments, and demographic and other data to help identify areas most at risk, then work with partner departments and organisations to promote evidence-based mitigation measures. As trusted professionals, they can engage with communities to provide information and guidance on how best to minimise health risks. Their role is crucial in ensuring initiatives are planned and implemented in the most appropriate way to benefit the people who need them most.

Transport is the largest greenhouse gas-emitting sector in the UK, accounting for 28% of total emissions.[26] It has been estimated that short car journeys of up to 16 kilometres are responsible for

40% of all emissions from vehicles.[27] Our dependence on cars reduces physical activity and contributes to obesity-related illness and deaths. Towns and cities can choose to establish alternatives to car journeys through 'active travel' such as cycling, walking and using electric buses, including ensuring that sufficient services exist for those unable to use active travel. A public health approach promotes to the local population the twin benefits of active travel – health improvement and reduced gas emissions.

'Green space' is an important element in mitigating the effects of climate change. Exposure to green space helps improve mood, reduces anxiety as well as lessens the risk of type 2 diabetes and cardiovascular disease.[28] 'Green exercise' or taking physical activity in green environments also benefits health. There are several environmental health benefits. For example, green space has been shown to reduce the likelihood of flooding, improve air quality and provide cooling and shade.[29] It has been estimated that £2.1 billion a year could be saved in healthcare costs if everyone in England had good access to green space.[30] Public health teams in local councils can promote the protection of existing green spaces and argue for increased green space in less-well off areas, as well as encouraging activities such as 'green walking' to improve health.

Health services

The UK's National Health Service (NHS), by its sheer size and reach across the population, is in an ideal position to lead by example on climate change and influence those with whom it comes into contact. It has one of the largest carbon profiles in the country and is energy intensive, responsible for 5% of the country's national greenhouse gas emissions.[31] It needs urgently to develop strategies to prepare for climate resilience and protect against risks in key areas such as water, waste and electricity supply. The NHS in England became the first healthcare system in the world in October 2020 to commit to a target to reduce carbon emissions (net zero by 2040).

The NHS could encourage its staff and patients to adopt habits that would be good for their health and for the planet. Moving away from diesel and petrol vehicles and towards active travel to lower emissions and reduce air pollution is one example. A public health approach also supports initiatives such as remote consulting, where appropriate clinically, to reduce unnecessary patient and staff travel.

The sustainable development special interest group of the Faculty of Public Health set out in 2021 key areas for action that public health practitioners can help health services with:

- Supporting patients to take a bigger role in managing their own health and health care such as having healthier diets which are more plant-based;
- Promoting active travel;
- Providing services where people need them (and avoid unnecessary travel);
- Streamlining care to minimise low value activity;
- Advising on impacts on health of overheating and cold so that temperatures in buildings are monitored and cool areas identified for staff and patient;.
- Advocating low-carbon alternatives to some medication, such as metered dose inhalers; reducing the impact of some anaesthetic agents which contain potent greenhouse gases;
- Advising on clinically and cost-effective alternatives to drug therapy fand promoting sustainable mental health;
- Adopting low carbon alternatives including using technologies with lower environmental impact and
- Minimising waste of medications, consumables and energy.[32]

The large part played by medicines and medical equipment should not be overlooked. One of the major shifts to date has been in the use of asthma inhalers, with more patients being treated using technology that provides effective treatment without contributing to build-up of greenhouse gases.[33] Public health input to commissioning and procurement can help increase the pace of change in this and other areas of clinical practice.

Air pollution

Air pollution is an important part of the climate health challenge because of the direct negative health impact of increased particulate matter and nitrogen dioxide in the air. These pollutants are also often produced alongside other greenhouse gases. Air pollution exacerbates asthma and chronic obstructive pulmonary disease. Long-term exposure can cause serious conditions such as chronic cardiovascular disease and lung cancer.[34] People at greatest risk of air pollution often live close to major roads or industrial plants, often in low-income households. Air pollution is, therefore, a cause of increased health inequalities. Reducing air pollution has benefits both for human health directly and for planetary health.

In the UK, it is estimated that air pollution is responsible for 28,000 to 36,000 excess deaths a year, mainly from respiratory and heart diseases, with the health and social care costs of air pollutants between 2017 and 2025 projected to be £1.6 billion.[35]

Air pollution originates mainly from human activities that use fossil fuels such as transport, industrial processes, farming, energy generation and domestic heating. Indoor air pollutants[36] include particulates[37] from domestic appliances (boilers, heaters, fires, stoves and ovens) which burn carbon-containing fuels that are not smoke-free such as coal, gas, coke, heating oil and wood). Tobacco smoke and second-hand smoke are also air pollutants.

Public health teams work with local authority planning and transport departments, as part of the development of sustainable towns and cities, to decrease the impact of air pollution locally. They can highlight and target for action those areas where air pollution is doing the greatest harm to residents. They can conduct evidence-based reviews on the impact of air pollution on the health of the local population. Action plans can address the most effective ways to reduce air pollution while also addressing health inequalities. Public health teams can provide public education to promote health, such as limiting strenuous activity when pollution is at its worst or reducing exposure to polluted outdoor air by closing external doors and windows facing busy streets.[38]

There is a close relationship between climate change and human health. Worsening environmental conditions drive health challenges and timely health-focused action helps mitigate those impacts. Public health voices are needed across continents to ensure these timely and effective actions if the opportunities for effective mitigation are not to be missed.

NOTES

1 An endemic disease is one that routinely occurs in an identified country. So, for example, the coronavirus causing COVID-19 is now endemic in most countries of the world; while malaria is endemic in tropical countries where anopheles mosquitoes thrive.

2 The links between antivaxxers and racism is well described in this article published in 2021: https://theconversation.com/the-inherent-racism-of-anti-vaxx-movements-163456

3 https://data.worldbank.org/indicator/SH.XPD.CHEX.GD.ZS

4 https://www.nice.org.uk/what-nice-does [accessed 4 December 2025]

5 A tertiary service is one that requires highly specialised medical staff and/or facilities, often found only in large teaching hospitals, which in the UK tend to be in cities

6 GAVI's description of war and public health may be found at: https://www.gavi.org/vaccineswork/wars-public-health-impacts-are-vast-tallying-them-difficult?gad_source=1&gad_campaignid=12319817265&gbraid=0AAAADibICPtDA5IoeoUz3eRpuySvamM1&gclid=CjwKCAiA55rJBhByEiwAFkY1QMixIRD3jb-dQo_yMBVgW2i4JCJJZnYvpBnUaTH4JD_fmB8hHh94dxoCjJwQAvD_BwE

7 https://commonslibrary.parliament.uk/research-briefings/sn04304/

8 For an objective description of what happened at Columbine see: https://www.britannica.com/event/Columbine-High-School-shootings [accessed 2 December 2025]

9 The Health Foundation 2025: https://www.health.org.uk/features-and-opinion/podcasts/ai-in-health-care-an-update-from-the-us

10 For details on Kaiser's seven principles of responsible use of AI, see: https://about.kaiserpermanente.org/news/ai-in-health-care-7-principles-of-responsible-use [accessed 26 November 2025]

11 https://www.gov.uk/government/news/new-commission-to-help-accelerate-nhs-use-of-ai

12 https://www.gov.uk/government/news/major-nhs-ai-trial-delivers-unprecedented-time-and-cost-savings

13 https://www.gov.uk/government/news/ai-to-be-trialled-at-unprecedented-scale-across-nhs-screening

14 The UK aims to reach net zero by 2050. https://unfccc.int/process-and-meetings/the-paris-agreement

15 https://www.nytimes.com/interactive/2025/11/07/climate/paris-agreement-climate.html

16 WHO, 12 October 2023, https://www.who.int/news-room/fact-sheets/detail/climate-change-and-health

17 WHO, 'Draft Global Action Plan on Climate Change and Health', 15 May 2025. https://apps.who.int/gb/ebwha/pdf_files/WHA78/A78_4Add2-en.pdf

18 https://www.who.int/news-room/fact-sheets/detail/climate-change-and-health, 12 October 2023.

19 https://ukhsa.blog.gov.uk/2023/12/11/11-things-to-know-about-the-health-effects-of-climate-change-report/

20 The Marmot Review of 2010 describes how nature contributes to both physical and mental health as well as encouraging social activity and reducing crime. Marmot, M., Goldblatt, P., Allen, J. et al., *Fair Society, Healthy Lives: The Marmot Review*, Institute of Health Equity 11 February 2010. https://www.gov.uk/research-for-development-outputs/fair-society-healthy-lives-the-marmot-review-strategic-review-of-health-inequalities-in-england-post-2010

21 https://assets.publishing.service.gov.uk/media/67fe2667694d57c6b1cf8d3c/AWHP_2025_to_2026.pdf

22 'UKSHA Incidence Response Roles', 15 January 2025. https://www.gov.uk/government/publications/emergency-preparedness-resilience-and-response-concept-of-operations/annexe-f-ukhsa-incident-response-roles

23 Stop or reduce carbon gases, especially carbon dioxide, being released into the atmosphere as the result of, for example the burning of fossil fuels.

24 Climate Change Act UK 2008. https://www.legislation.gov.uk/ukpga/2008/27/contents

25 'Fuel poverty' relates to households that must spend a high proportion of their household income to keep their home at a reasonable temperature. https://commonslibrary.parliament.uk/research-briefings/cbp-8730/ 14 April 2025.

26 Climate Change and Health: Applying All Our Health, 18 May 2022. https://www.gov.uk/government/publications/climate-change-applying-all-our-health/climate-and-health-applying-all-our-health

27 Association of Directors of Public Health, Public Health's Role in Tackling Climate Change', 18 January 2024. https://www.adph.org.uk/2024/01/public-healths-role-in-tackling-climate-change/

28 Climate Change and Health: Applying All Our Health, 18 May 2022. https://www.gov.uk/government/publications/climate-change-applying-all-our-health/climate-and-health-applying-all-our-health

29 Kingsley, M., 'Commentary Climate Change, Health And Green Space Co-Benefits', *Health Promotion and Chronic Diseease Prevention in Canada*, 39(4):131–35, April 2019. https://pmc.ncbi.nlm.nih.gov/articles/PMC6553580/

30 Climate Change and Health: Applying All Our Health, 18 May 2022. https://www.gov.uk/government/publications/climate-change-applying-all-our-health/climate-and-health-applying-all-our-health

31 Climate Change and Health: Applying All Our Health, 18 May 2022. https://www.gov.uk/government/publications/climate-change-applying-all-our-health/climate-and-health-applying-all-our-health

32 Faculty of Public Health Special Interest Group – Sustainable Development. https://www.fph.org.uk/media/3128/a9-fph-sig-towards-a-net-zero-carbon-nhs-final.pdf

33 NICE, 'Asthma Inhalers and Climate Change'. https://www.nice.org.uk/guidance/ng245/resources/patient-decision-aid-on-asthma-inhalers-and-climate-change-bts-nice-sign-pdf-13558151917

34 Office for Health Improvement and Disparities, 'Air Pollution: Applying All Our Health', 28 February 2022. https://www.gov.uk/government/publications/air-pollution-applying-all-our-health/air-pollution-applying-all-our-health

35 British Medical Association, 'Climate Change and Air Pollution', 7 December 2023. https://www.bma.org.uk/what-we-do/population-health/protecting-people-from-threats-to-health/climate-change-and-air-pollution

36 A pollutant is a substance that pollutes something, especially water or the atmosphere.

37 Particulates are microscopic particles of solid or liquid matter suspended in the air – they are often pollutants.

38 Office for Health Improvement and Disparities, 'Air Pollution; Applying All Our Health', updated 28 February 2022. https://www.gov.uk/government/publications/air-pollution-applying-all-our-health/air-pollution-applying-all-our-health

SOURCES ACCESSED IN COMPILING THIS CHAPTER AND FURTHER READING

EXAMPLE OF GLOBAL POLITICS OF HEALTH – TACKLING MALARIA

CDC, 2024, 'Strategies for Reducing Malaria's Global Impact'. https://www.cdc.gov/malaria/php/public-health-strategy/index.html [accessed 4 December 2025]

WAR, CONFLICT

GAVI's description of war and public health, 18 October 2024, 'War's Public Health Impacts Are Vast'. https://www.gavi.org/vaccineswork/wars-public-health-impacts-are-vast-tallying-them-difficult?gad_source=1&gad_campaignid=12319817265&gbraid=0AAAADibICPtDA5IoeoUz3eRpuySvamM1&gclid=CjwKCAiA55rJBhByEiwAFkY1QMixIRD3jb-dQo_yMBVgW2i4JCJJZnYvpBnUaTH4JD_fmB8hHh94dxoCjJwQAvD_BwE

ARTIFICIAL INTELLIGENCE

Coursera free open access short course. 'Introduction to Using Generative AI in Public Health', Johns Hopkins University. https://www.coursera.org/learn/generative-ai-to-improve-public-health [accessed 4 December 2025].

Association of Directors of Public Health, 'AI and Health', King's Festival of Artificial Intelligence, 21 May 2025. https://www.adph.org.uk/networks/london/events/ai-and-health-kings-festival-of-artificial-intelligence-2/

Faculty of Public Health, Artificial Intelligence and Digital Public Health Special Interest Group (SIG). https://www.fph.org.uk/policy-advocacy/special-interest-groups/artificial-intelligence-digital-public-health-sig/

Glasgow Centre for Population Health, 'The Potential of Artificial Intelligence (AI) within Public Health and Healthcare Systems', April 2025. https://www.gcph.co.uk/latest/publications/1240-the-potential-of-artificial-intelligence-ai-within-public-health-and-healthcare-systems

GOV.UK, 'Press Release: AI to be trialled at unprecedented scale across NHS screening', 22 September 2025. https://www.gov.uk/government/news/ai-to-be-trialled-at-unprecedented-scale-across-nhs-screening

Health AI (the Global Agency for Responsible AI in Health), 'Leadership and Governance'. https://healthai.agency/leadership-governance/

Intelligent Transport Systems UK, 'Vivacity's AI Powered Data Insights Help Sheffield City Council Boost Air Quality', 5 September 2023. https://www.its-uk.org/vivacitys-ai-powered-data-insights-help-sheffield-city-council-boost-air-quality/

NHS England, 'AI Knowledge Repository'. For case studies and examples: https://digital.nhs.uk/services/ai-knowledge-repository

The Alan Turing Institute, 'Public Health AI Debate: Is It Time for Public Health to Shift Focus to the Individual?', July 2025. https://www.turing.ac.uk/events/public-health-ai-debate-it-time-public-health-shift-focus-individual

CLIMATE CHANGE SOURCES FOR THIS CHAPTER

Association of Directors of Public Health, 'Public Health's Role in Tackling Climate Change', 18 January 2024. https://www.adph.org.uk/2024/01/public-healths-role-in-tackling-climate-change/

British Medical Association, 'Climate Change and Air Pollution', 7 December 2023. https://www.bma.org.uk/what-we-do/population-health/protecting-people-from-threats-to-health/climate-change-and-air-pollution

Faculty of Public Health, 'Resources on Climate Change and Health'. https://www.fph.org.uk/policy-advocacy/special-interest-groups/sustainable-development-sig/resources-on-climate-change-and-health/

Goniewicz, K., Burkle, F.M. and Khorram-Manesh, A., 'Transforming Global Public Health: Climate Collaboration, Political Challenges, and Systemic Change', *Journal of Infection and Public Health*, 18(1), January 2025. https://www.sciencedirect.com/science/article/pii/S1876034124003496

Kreslake, J.M., Sarfaty, M., Roser-Renouf, C. et al., 'The Critical Roles of Health Professional in Climate Change Prevention and Preparedness', *American Journal of Public Health*, April 2018, 108 (Suppl 2): S68–69. https://pmc.ncbi.nlm.nih.gov/articles/PMC5922192/#:~:text=Local%2C%20state%2C%20and%20federal%20public,illness%20exacerbated%20by%20climate%20change

Royal Society for Public Health, *Public Health 2040: Health Protection in a Warming World*, 13 September 2024. https://www.rsph.org.uk/media/filer_public/a6/4f/a64f5d76-6df3-4b1c-b086-148baa3c3f6e/ph2040-health-protection-in-a-warming-world-briefing.pdf

Sim, F. and Wright J., *Working in Public Health – Choosing the Right Career*, 2nd Edition, Routledge, 2024.

GENERAL READING ON CLIMATE CHANGE

Griffiths, J., Rao, M., Adshead, F. and Thorpe, A. (eds) *The Health Practitioner's Guide to Climate Change – Diagnosis And Cure*, Earthscan, 2009.

Climate Change Committee: https://www.theccc.org.uk/climate-action/

NHS Open Access E-Learning module about Climate Change for Health and Care professionals: https://portal.e-lfh.org.uk/Component/Details/603166

IN CONCLUSION

You have reached the end, and we hope you now know more about the world of public health – what it is, what it contributes to our health and wellbeing, why it is important.

We have covered the history and waves of public health development from the nineteenth century through to the present day with changes and adaptations according to population health need. On the way, we have explained key terms in public health and what the discipline of public health entails – knowledge, competences, experience. We have described the workforce, how it is trained, the functions it carries out and the desire to protect the population from ill-health, promote good health and reduce inequalities which unite it. Lastly, we have aimed to present some of the continuing and future challenges facing those working in public health along with ways they can make a contribution.

There have been many successes and achievements since the middle of the nineteenth century. Yet existing problems facing population health continue to be stubborn to manage whilst new problems emerge. For many issues, there are competing interests, at the very least from the commercial sector.

Tackling these issues will require a concerted effort from governments as much as from those working in public health, locally, nationally and internationally, as well as from the population at large. We will need an increasing, capable, flexible and sufficiently numerous work force to meet these challenges.

We have not speculated on the future and what the next wave in public health development might be as we head towards the middle of the twenty-first century. How different does it need to be in

DOI: 10.4324/9781003779902-17

the face of an increasing complex and unpredictable world? Those working in public health will need to look to innovation and more interdependence with others if we are to find satisfactory solutions on a large scale.[1] Another proposition is ecological public health, which integrates the material, biological, social, and cultural aspects of public health and links it with evidence, policy and practice.[2]

What is certain is that the world of public health will never be dull, its work never finished.

NOTES

1 Hanlon, P., Carlisle, S., Hannah, M., Reilly, D. and Lyon, A., 'Making the Case for a 'Fifth Wave' in Public Health', *Public Health*, 125(1): 30–36, January 2011. https://www.sciencedirect.com/science/article/abs/pii/S0033350610003197

2 'Ecological Public Health: The 21st Century's Big Idea? An Essay by Tim Lang and Geof Rayner', BMJ, 345:e5466, 21 August 2012. https://www.bmj.com/content/345/bmj.e5466.full

LIST OF ABBREVIATIONS (UK USAGE)

A&E	Accident and Emergency
AI	Artificial Intelligence
AGM	Annual General Meeting
AIDS	Acquired Immunodeficiency Syndrome
ASH	Action on Smoking and Health
APHA	American Public Health Association
ATACH	Alliance for Transformative Action on Climate and Health
BMA	British Medical Association
BMJ	British Medical Journal
CDS	Communicable Diseases
CDC	Centers for Disease Control and Prevention (USA)
CSR	Corporate Social Responsibility
DHSC	Department of Health and Social Care
DSPH	Directors of Public Health
Dte GHS	Directorate General of Health Services
ECDC	European Centre for Disease Prevention and Control
EHESP	Ecole des Hautes Etudes en Santé Publique
EEHP	Extreme Events and Health Protection
FCTC	(WHO) Framework Convention on Tobacco Control
FDA	Food and Drug Administration
FPH	Faculty of Public Health
GCSE	General Certificate of Secondary Education
GP	General Medical Practitioner
HCNA	Health Care Needs Assessment
HNA	Health Needs Assessment
HIA	Health Impact Assessment

HIC	Higher Income Countries
HIV	Human Immunodeficiency Viruses
HPV	Human papillomavirus
IHR	International Health Regulations
ILO	International Labour Organization
LAQM	Local Air Quality Management
LIC	Low-Income Countries
LMICS	Low- and Middle-Income Countries
LNHO	League of Nations Health Organization
LSHTM	London School of Hygiene and Tropical Medicine
MHRA	Medicines and Healthcare products Regulatory Agency
MERS	Middle East Respiratory Syndrome
MMR	Mumps, Measles and Rubella
MOOC	Massive Open Online Course
MSA	Master Settlement Agreement
MOH	Medical Officer of Health
MUP	Minimum Unit Pricing
NCMP	National Child Measurement Programme
NCDS	Non-communicable Diseases
NGO	Non-Governmental Organisation
NHBHE	National Board of Public Health Examiners, USA
NHS	National Health Service
NICE	National Institute of Health and Care Excellence
NRT	Nicotine Replacement Therapy
OHID	Office for Health Improvement and Disparities
PPE	Personal Protective Equipment
PROMS	Patient Reported Outcome Measures
RCT	Randomised Controlled Trial
PHSCC	US Public Health Service Commissioned Corps
RCP	Royal College of Physicians
RBM	Roll Back Malaria
RPI	Retail Price Index
SARS	Severe Acute Respiratory Syndrome
SIDS	Sudden Infant Death Syndrome
SMS	Short Message Service
SRIA	Strategic Research and Innovation Agenda
UK	United Kingdon
UKHSA	UK Health Security Agency
UN	United Nations

UNRAA	United National Relief and Rehabilitation Administration
UPF	Ultra Processed Food
USA	United States of America
VCS	Voluntary and Community Services
WHO	World Health Organization

INDEX

Note: page numbers followed by n refer to notes.

For Product Safety Concerns and Information please contact our EU representative GPSR@taylorandfrancis.com
Taylor & Francis Verlag GmbH, Kaufingerstraße 24, 80331 München, Germany

www.ingramcontent.com/pod-product-compliance
Ingram Content Group UK Ltd.
Pitfield, Milton Keynes, MK11 3LW, UK
UKHW022344190926
475702UK00015B/2085

* 9 7 8 1 0 3 2 8 3 4 7 1 9 *